Dementia and the Advance Directive

Marcia Sokolowski

Dementia and the Advance Directive

Lessons from the Bedside

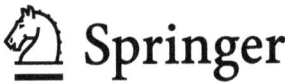 Springer

Marcia Sokolowski, Ph.D
Faculty of Medicine
Department of Medicine
University of Toronto
Toronto, ON, Canada

Centre for Health
Humanism and Society
Ben Gurion University of the Desert
Beer-Sheva, Israel

Baycrest Health Sciences
Toronto, ON, Canada

ISBN 978-3-030-10154-1   ISBN 978-3-319-72083-8   (eBook)
https://doi.org/10.1007/978-3-319-72083-8

Printed on acid-free paper

This Springer imprint is published by Springer Nature
The registered company is Springer International Publishing AG
The registered company address is: Gewerbestrasse 11, 6330 Cham, Switzerland

Disclaimer

The content in this book is provided for general information only, and is neither medical nor legal advice. If you have questions, please consult a professional advisor in your jurisdiction, as the terms referred to in the book may be called something different.

Preface

As both a clinical psychologist and a clinical ethicist, I have been fascinated with the topic of dementia and the topic of advance directives. The lenses I peer through in the writing of this book, in bringing these topics together, are in nature both philosophical (and ethics based) and psychological, bridging both my professional and academic careers.

This book is based upon a composite of multiple ethics cases over many years in a variety of settings and reflects my almost twenty-years practice in the role of medical ethicist as well as theories of ethics important to the presentation of the cases. These composite case studies depict very interesting and challenging moral issues arising in a variety of healthcare facilities in Ontario, Canada. The cases have been created as composites for privacy and confidentiality reasons. While identifying descriptors of persons have been removed, the ethical topics I raise represent common themes and dilemmas I have encountered. These are three in-depth altered and amalgamated cases created to depict the type of cases that can be found to be ethically unsettling, and I address approaches to resolving the moral conundrums that arise in these incredibly complex situations. In addition to inviting the reader inside real healthcare organizations, I lay bare a description and assessment of the dynamics of the interdisciplinary healthcare teams and the dynamics of the families who are grappling to best serve their loved ones. After each case study, I apply the concepts I introduced in the beginning of the book to the case study at hand, thus integrating theory with a case-based approach. I employ a question-and-answer format that I believe is very user-friendly and provides for thought provoking and accessible learning experiences, as I walk readers through my approach at tackling these complicated and realistic advance directive situations. Additionally, I consistently emphasize the complexity and individuality of each case, suggesting an updated framework and thought process when dealing with the implementation and execution of advance directives.

Note that I use a general term, "advance directive". While this term is not generally used in Ontario, I employ it here to cover the broad range of terms such as written wishes, powers of attorney, living wills and others, which may be used elsewhere. It will be important for the reader to know which terms actually apply in the jurisdiction where they live; and more importantly, to understand whether a written document that expresses a person's wishes can be relied on to ground informed consent; and whether it must be interpreted either by a substitute decision-maker (another term that may vary) or can be relied on directly by a health practitioner. Please read "advance directive" with these caveats.

At first, I was encouraged by the idea that an advance directive could provide a much needed voice to the person with dementia. Then I questioned the utility of this idea—could this really be so? And if so, is this really a good thing? I argue that we need to be wary of using advance directives with the dementia population, at least in the way they are currently used. Although advance directives have been presented to the public as the ideal way to avoid problems when it comes to understanding the wishes that form the basis for medical decisions for previously capable patients, they do not always work as well as intended.

I challenge the more traditional conceptualizations of autonomy, competency, and informed consent and suggest they be tweaked and better understood. I offer alternatives that I believe align better with the realities of persons' experiences living with dementia. Rather than taking the age-old approach of using the concept of personhood to discuss and resolve the problems in these cases, I argue that our notions of autonomy and informed consent are not only ill developed and ill understood by the healthcare communities, but they are also not fluid enough to be of real help in most situations. This I believe leaves a great opening for a new discussion about autonomy and informed consent, including how advance directive use can be improved via defining autonomy as the ability to create and hold onto wishes in regard to values that matter most to the person in question. I think the introduction of values is another one of my unique contributions since most of the discussion of autonomy and competency does not place enough weight on values.

At the end of the book, I list more specific conclusions and practical recommendations, which include, but are not limited to, improving education for all people involved (patients when writing advance directives, family members (i.e., substitute decision-makers) when interpreting them, staff when helping substitute decision-makers to understand their role in the interpretation of them); treating advance directives as only one, defeasible, piece of information about the patient's wishes; and coming to recognize and give weight to the current interests and concerns of a patient with dementia.

It is my hope that this book will be of interest and benefit to academic audiences, interdisciplinary clinicians, and the general public who is interested in learning more about/compiling their own advance directives.

Toronto, ON, Canada   Marcia Sokolowski

Acknowledgements

I want to express my deepest gratitude to Tim Kenyon and Mary Jane Dykeman for their wisdom and collegiality; to Richard Lansing and Caitlin Prim of Springer Nature for extending this exciting opportunity to me and championing this important topic; to my family, Howard Sokolowski, Linda Frum and Honey Apter for unconditional caring and support, and to my son Corey Sokolowski for being my brilliant and best teacher; and always, to my late parents Henry and Eva Sokolowski, who believed in me, and whose memory lights my path every day.

Contents

Chapter 1
Introduction

Setting the Stage

Barack Obama became the first US President to announce publicly that he had a living will (also known as an advance directive, among other terms which vary from one jurisdiction to another), and he encouraged his fellow Americans to do the same. On July 28, 2009, he spoke the following words at a town hall meeting: "So I actually think it's a good idea to have a living will. I'd encourage everybody to get one. I have one; Michelle has one. And we hope we don't have to use it for a long time, but I think it's something that is sensible."[1]

But is Obama correct? Is an advance directive a useful decision-making tool to have when one has Alzheimer's, for example? I hope to answer this perplexing question in this book. At first blush many people (including myself) think having one could stand them in good stead. Allow me to explain.

Most people shudder at the thought of having a dementia. Alzheimer's, the most common type, is often regarded as a fate worse than death and depicted as a disease that robs persons of their selves. Many fear that, as a result of technological advances, they will be kept alive much longer than they would like to be, suffering from the indignities of old age and dementia. They worry that the protective instincts of medical professionals or sheer bureaucratic inertia might result in prolonging their lives under conditions they consider hellish from their current perspectives. Or perhaps their loved ones or legal guardians would be not so well intentioned and would make decisions according to their own best interests and not according to those of their relatives with dementia.

This is where the idea of an *advance directive* (otherwise known as instructions regarding healthcare treatment choices projected into a future time of incapacity)

---

[1] Conolly, Ceci. "Obama takes personal approach in AARP speech," The Washington Post, July 29, 2009.

© Springer International Publishing AG 2018
M. Sokolowski, *Dementia and the Advance Directive*,
https://doi.org/10.1007/978-3-319-72083-8_1

can become very alluring.[2] It is often seen as the answer to one of our biggest worries—that we will have no control over our lives when we are old, sick, and possibly suffering miserably with a dementia. The worst nightmare seems to be that we will have lost the right to say "no" to life-sustaining treatment. This grave concern, and sometimes an associated one that we will become a burden to our children in our old age, motivates people to complete what is known as an advance directive.[3]

In this book on advance directives, it is my intention to demonstrate that it is far from enjoying perfect health these days. My question is whether it is worth resuscitating the advance directive or is it time to pull the plug on it? In the following chapters, I will lay out various theories, strategies, and case studies in order to consider the strengths and weaknesses that exist.

My writings are based upon my experiences of being an ethicist within several healthcare facilities in Ontario, Canada, for almost two decades. While the case studies I present are based in this context, this book is aimed at a broader audience, including Western democratic populations, such as North America; Central, Northern, and Western Europe (including the United Kingdom); New Zealand; and Australia.[4] My purpose in the following chapters is to present several anonymized and composite case studies that reflect a broad spectrum of data from my clinical consultation practice. These case studies are representative of the kind of vexing, challenging cases that keep me up into the wee hours of the night.

As an ethicist one of my duties is to provide consultation to staff, patients, and families, dealing with moral issues. Ultimately, decisions are supposed to be made that are in the best interests of the patients we care for. Often ethical issues arise as moral dilemmas when there is difficulty knowing what is the right thing to do in relation to particular ethical principles. As it often happens, there may not be one right thing to do, and/or we may never really know if the decision was *the* right one. Nonetheless, as moral agents of a community, we feel an obligation to try to do what is right.[5]

---

[2] Advance directive is also known as a *living will* or *directive*. As noted, while "advance directive" is not a term used in Ontario, I use it here to encompass the wishes of the patient regarding future healthcare, which could be captured verbally, or in writing in a power of attorney or other document. It will be important for readers to know the terms used in their own jurisdictions; and to understand whom the wishes guide – whether they are to be interpreted by a substitute decision-maker (substitute, proxy or other term), or whether a health practitioner may act directly on the wish.

[3] The concept of the living will became enshrined in US legislation in the 1990s following the high profile cases of Karen Quinlan and Nancy Cruzan. Jane Seymour and Gillian Horne, "Advance Care Planning for the end of life: an overview" in Advance Care Planning in End of Life Care, ed. Keri Thomas and Ben Lobo (Oxford: Oxford University Press, 2011), 18.

[4] Specific laws pertaining to advance directives and powers of attorney may and often do differ between these countries and within jurisdictions of each particular country. No formal requirements exist for advance directives or living wills in Ontario - no Ontario statute exists that makes reference to them. Wishes made about future care including treatment can be incorporated into a legal Power of Attorney for Personal Care document that does have formal requirements.

[5] These discussions do not occur in a vacuum. Healthcare organizations are complex systems within themselves, and there are always larger social and political factors influencing the kinds of

In democratic societies a high value is placed on individuals' right to determine (within prescribed limits) what is right for them or in their own best interests. Individuals have the right to make their own choices and to decide and act in accordance with how they choose to live their lives, as long as they are considered to be capable to do so.[6] Respect for this right, reflected in the principle of autonomy, is foundational to the moral and legal practice of medicine in democratic societies.

Over the past few decades, the pendulum has swung significantly from a dominant paternalistic approach (protection of patients, assumptions that the healthcare providers know best what their patients need) to a greater respect for autonomy of patients (the patients' right to consent to, or refuse, medical treatment).[7] While most healthcare organizations try to provide care that takes into account the patients' choices, wishes, and interests, the concept of autonomy remains rather vague.

Sadly, many patients have medical conditions that prevent them from being able to express their wishes. Sometimes they may not be considered mentally capable to consent to or refuse treatment due to an existing dementia, such as Alzheimer's.[8] This neurological disease is progressive, eventually resulting in death, usually within 10 years. Difficulties with memory and other cognitive deficits generally increase over time, although the overall decline is peppered with instances of clearer thoughts and memories. Given the aging population we serve, many patients have additional health problems that require decisions to be made.

The Advance Directive

Capable adults are allowed to provide instructions about their healthcare choices in case of future incapacity. Capable adults may also appoint an individual (or individuals) to speak on their behalf at such times. These designated persons are called

---

care that can be offered and how that care is distributed. Healthcare policies and guidelines are driven by the organization's mission, vision, and codes of conduct, and there are many different types of healthcare personnel involved in decision-making and the delivery of care.

[6] This right is encoded in democratic legislation. For example, see Ontario's *Health Care Consent Act, 1996*, S.O. c.2, s. A., p.1.4. Additionally, please note that while the term adopted is *"capable"* per the Ontario legislation, the term *competent* may also be used and is interchangeable unless otherwise noted.

[7] Alfred Simon, "Historical Review of Advance Directives," in *Advance Directives*, ed. Peter Lack, Nikola Biller-Andorno and Susanne Brauer (Springer Press New York, 2014), 3. However, there are some limitations to this kind of autonomous freedom we speak about. For one thing, patients have no right to receive absolutely any treatment they wish. The healthcare practitioners have no duty to provide an ineffective treatment and also have a duty to not do harm. See J.M. Atkinson, Advance Directives in Mental Health: Theory, Practice and Ethics (London: Jessica Kingsley Publishers, 2007): 74.

[8] While all dementias have some commonality, I am restricting my focus to only dementia of the Alzheimer's type, the most common one.

substitute decision-makers (herein to be called SDMs), or may have another name in other jurisdictions, such as "proxies".[9]

Many people verbally express their wishes to their loved ones. A smaller number put them in writing. As a result of some recent landmark cases (where there was a great deal of conflict ensuing about whether to withdraw life-sustaining treatment from people in vegetative states), there has been a rapid increase in people completing their advance directives. Basically, its future use is mainly for SDMs (or medical professionals in some jurisdictions) to help guide medical decision-making. When you write an advance directive, you are (allegedly) projecting your medical treatment wishes into the future. This document will speak for you through the voices of your SDMs (or in some jurisdictions – not Ontario - your healthcare practitioners) if you are unable to do so yourself.

The statements in advance directives regarding one's wishes for future treatment are often framed in general terms. Occasionally, specific details are given regarding the conditions that should be in place in order for a specific treatment wish to be complied with.[10] Documents are often downloaded from legal websites, and there may (or may not) be a great deal of thought put into the writing of them. Wishes might be impulsively scribbled onto a cocktail napkin or more thoroughly contemplated and formally documented. Sometimes lawyers are involved who offer additional input as to the benefits and consequences of writing a directive. Sometimes loved ones participate in the process. The directive may be regularly updated or forgotten about.

There are a number of potential benefits in creating an advance directive. Some people feel great relief and lessened anxiety believing they have taken some control over their future lives. They might feel gratified to think that they have relieved their loved ones from making difficult decisions on their behalf. Their loved ones may share this relief as well as experience a sense of comfort believing they have honored their loved ones' end of life wishes. Having an advance directive might decrease moral distress among and between family members and healthcare professionals that might arise from conflict about healthcare decision-making. Nonetheless many problems that we will discuss further on in the book still occur and they will be detailed in the upcoming chapters.

The important thing is that at a future time when you are deemed to be incapable, if your expressed treatment wishes in an advance directive are known to be your most recent capable ones, they might carry as much legal weight as if you were capable of uttering them at that time.[11] So be careful what you wish for!

---

[9] Many people designate an SDM to speak on their behalf, regardless of whether or not they have an advance directive. In Ontario the legal term for such a person is *attorney for personal care*. If there is no legal attorney for personal care, then in Ontario there is a hierarchical ranking of persons from which a selection is identified, eligible to fulfill that role. The designation of SDM is used in these circumstances. However, for simplicity's sake, I will use the term SDM to refer as well to the attorney for personal care.

[10] The term *treatment wishes* is used both to denote treatments the author of the directive wishes to receive and treatments the author wishes to refuse in the future.

[11] Assuming that you were deemed capable at the time you wrote your advance directive.

When I first started working as a medical ethicist, I thought having an advance directive would likely be very beneficial. I took great comfort in the idea of being able to control now what my future "me" will experience. Several years of clinical practice have passed, and my previous enthusiasm has been largely tempered. No doubt there are situations where having an advance directive might serve me well.[12] However, I am quite concerned that the same directive that now allows me the freedom to decide for myself could in the future be experienced by me as imprisonment. That is, my future self will be chained to the wishes of my former self.[13]

So we already have a raft of disturbing questions. For example, what if I change my mind but can't express myself clearly? What if I'm not taken seriously because I'm old and I have a dementia and my current wish seems strange or dumb to them? What if a cure for my condition will be available very soon, but I've asked for no treatment under circumstances that exist *now*?[14] What if my children who are my attorneys for personal care don't agree on how to interpret my wishes? It's as easy to see problems with advance directives as it is to see their promise.[15] As I proceed with this discussion, these problems will become sharper and still others will emerge. Because the problems depicted and the arguments I make are case-driven and cumulative, certain elements will recur in each chapter. I will, however, attempt to show at each stage how the immediate considerations relate to those already raised in previous chapters. I think it bears repeating that while I focus on Ontario with regard to the case studies, laws, professional practices, and standards I discuss, many of my observations and claims could potentially be generalized to other North American, United Kingdom, Australian, and New Zealand regions as well as in Central, Northern, and Western Europe where advance directives also exist.

As will be evidenced, definitions employed in some core domains of law (e.g., executing a power of attorney for personal care, etc.) end up determining or at least skewing the interpretations of autonomy, competence, and other core concepts that are at stake when we consider the best way to safeguard the rights and dignity of persons with Alzheimer's. Legally useful conceptions of capacity and autonomy in these core domains do not translate easily into morally defensible conceptions in the cases of advance directives among the dementia population. It is plausible that parallel problems (related to overgeneralized concepts of overidealized agency—issues to be discussed later) will arise virtually everywhere—after all, working from precedent and generalizing from core cases is how law works, in the absence of special

---

[12] Later I will broaden the scope to include the larger network of family and professional staff when considering the benefits and burdens of having an advance directive.

[13] Simon, 11

[14] Robert Olick, "On the Scope and Limits of Advance Directives and Prospective Autonomy," Advance Directives, ed. Peter Lack, Nikola Biller-Andorno, and Susanne Brauer (New York: Springer, 2014) 67. Olick considers the situation when there has been a "radical change in circumstances from those previously contemplated by the patient" and asserts the argument that there would be justified reason to override the patient's directive previously requesting refusal of treatment.

[15] Simon, 12

reasons to have domain-specific exceptions. The problems I diagnose, or close ana-
logues of them, are likely to arise in any legally and medically similar context.

In theory the advance directive seems like a good idea. But like other good ideas,
in reality, it is quite flawed—at least in the way an advance directive is used now
today. However, before we agree to pull the plug, there might be some useful or
constructive ways to revive it. The problems will become clearer through the cases
I present. What I want to do here is to expose the complexities and challenges
advance directives raise and to identify a broad range of predicaments that arise out
of their use with the Alzheimer's dementia population I work with. Some of these
predicaments are more problematic than others. Some are general to all situations,
some more specific. By laying them out at least, we can identify where the more
serious issues lie and determine if we can do anything to either solve their problems
or at least minimize them. Perhaps it is premature to pull the plug on the advance
directive after all!

Alzheimer's Dementia

Now that the reader has a basic introduction to the advance directive, it is imperative
to provide a brief overview of Alzheimer's dementia. The Latin word "dementia"
was first used in first-century Rome and stems from the word *demens* meaning "out
of one's mind."[16] In North America as well as in many other Western countries, a
commonly held view of Alzheimer's dementia is that it is a disease that robs persons
of their selves, mainly owing to progressive loss of memory.[17] It would be hard to
identify any other disease feared today (at least in North America) with equal inten-
sity and automatically associated with loss of personal identity.

As I mentioned, the most common form of dementia in older people is the
Alzheimer's type where characteristically there is a declining function among a
number of intellectual abilities.[18] There may be problems with aspects of language
(including grammatically correct sentences), understanding concepts, making good
judgments, doing simple calculations, organizing series of body movements, and
remembering recent events.[19] Changes in personality and behavior are noted as

---

[16] Carmelo Aquilina and Julian C. Hughes, "The Return of the Living Dead: Agency Lost and
Found?" in *Dementia: Mind, Meaning, and the Person*, ed. Julian C. Hughes, Stephen J. Louw, and
Steven R. Sabat (Oxford: Oxford University Press, 2006), 143. Also see Herskovits who speaks of
the concept of Alzheimer's disease as a "monsterizing of senility." Elizabeth Herskovits,
"Struggling over Subjectivity: Debates about the 'Self' and Alzheimer's Disease," *Medical
Anthropology Quarterly* 9, no. 2(1995): 153.

[17] Prominent theorist Rebecca Dresser supports the argument that memory loss contributes to a loss
of self in patients with severe dementia. See Rebecca Dresser, "Dworkin on Dementia: Elegant
Theory, Questionable Policy," *Hastings Centre Report* 25, no. 6 (1995): 35.

[18] L.K. Fellows, "Competency and Consent in Dementia," *Journal of American Geriatrics Society*
46, no.7 (1998): 922.

[19] Steven R. Sabat, "Capacity for Decision-Making in Alzheimer's Disease: Selfhood, Positioning

well.[20] The disease is progressive and, as mentioned, usually results in death about 10 years later. Typically the disease is described as being in one of three stages, mild, moderate, or severe, although progression from one to the next is not necessarily linear. A definitive diagnosis relies upon both a clinical picture and findings on autopsy. There is no known cure presently.

In my clinical experience, I am hard-pressed to recall ethics-based discussions that did not directly or indirectly refer in some way, shape or form, to the notion of autonomy, especially in the context of declining functional abilities of those diagnosed with Alzheimer's. The relationship between this disease and autonomy is not so straightforward, at least in my opinion, for a variety of reasons. The next section provides some insight into what I mean by this.

Autonomy

Bioethics, the study of moral issues in the field of medicine, emerged as a distinct discipline during the past four decades, owing much to the work of bioethicists Thomas Beauchamp and James Childress. They developed an approach to bioethics whereby four universal moral principles can be applied to particular ethical problems. These principles are autonomy[21], non-maleficence (do no harm), beneficence (do good), and justice.[22] There is no evidence that Beauchamp and Childress considered any one principle to be of higher value than another. However, in current healthcare practice, at least in North America, the principle of autonomy usually reigns as supreme.[23]

In the forthcoming section on "Informed Consent," we will see how autonomy is narrowly defined when it comes to medical decision-making and understood in the

---

and Semiotic People," *Australian and New Zealand Journal of Psychiatry* 39, no. 11-12 (Nov 2005): 1030.

[20] Pam Sailors, "Autonomy, Benevolence, and Alzheimer's Disease," *Cambridge Quarterly of Healthcare Ethics* 10 (2001): 184.

[21] F. Baylis, J. Downie, B. Hoffmaster, S. Sherwin, ed., *Health Care Ethics in Canada*, 2nd ed. (Toronto: Nelson, 2004), 7. "Autonomy" and "respect for autonomy" are terms loosely associated with several ideas, such as privacy, voluntariness, self-mastery, choosing freely, choosing one's own moral position, and accepting responsibility for one's choices.

[22] T.I. Beauchamp and J.F. Childress, *Principles of Biomedical Ethics* (New York: Oxford University Press, 2001): 121. Also see Susan Dodds, "Choice and Control in Feminist Bioethics," in *Relational Autonomy: Feminist Perspectives on Autonomy, Agency and the Social Self*, ed. Catriona Mackenzie and Natalie Stoljar (Oxford University Press US, 2000), 215.

[23] There is however much controversy among bioethicists today about the justification of its elevated status. As referred to earlier, the privileged role that autonomy holds today in healthcare ethics is also understood as a backlash against what is perceived to be a largely paternalistic model of medical decision-making of the past where doctors and other healthcare providers are deemed to be the experts who generally made the decisions themselves according to their patients' best interests (as they perceived them to be).

context of actions as opposed to what it means to be an autonomous person.[24] We will also note how the concept of autonomy and concept of competence (or capacity) are often understood to be interchangeable. There may have been good historic reasons for this to have evolved, both from a legal and clinical practice point of view. However, the unfortunate results are that most patients with dementia will at some point in time be inappropriately stripped of their rights to participate in decision-making matters that are important to them, because they will be deemed to be incapable, (and thus nonautonomous) and will be treated as persons whose ideas, values, beliefs, and interests do not count.[25] I will argue, instead, that we ought to think of autonomous persons as ones who have the ability to create or hold onto wishes and values that matter to them.

It may seem that speaking of wishes and values (and preferences and desires) blurs some important distinctions. Certainly there are important psychological and moral-theoretic differences among these states. Nevertheless, I sometimes refer to them interchangeably. I set the distinction aside for the following reason: I think my argument will show that we owe greater deference to (in the most general sense) the present psychological states of persons with dementia even if we only consider the states that seem most psychologically basic, and which they least controversially can be said to possess, such as desires. If it turns out that they can also be properly said to have arguably more complex and morally loaded states, such as *values* that are reflected in those desires, then the case I will make for increased deference would only be stronger.

In Chap. 3, I claim that many persons with dementia are still capable of having autonomy,[26] and, as an example, I present the case of Mrs. Black. I will also discuss the importance of viewing autonomy as fluctuating, and not necessarily absolute, but rather partial nor fixed over time. Additionally, I endorse the value of understanding autonomy within a relational framework.[27] Others in the patients' world can "step in" to try to assist patients with expressing their values in meaningful ways. For example, patients might be holding onto important values but have trouble communicating them. Others can try to discern what values and interests the patients are trying to convey so that current medical decisions can be made to cohere with them. The case of Mr. White in Chap. 4 illustrates these concepts and how they can be practically applied.

I earlier alluded to the idea that autonomy and informed consent are closely linked. The next section will hopefully shed further light on the relationship between the two.

---

[24] I strongly prefer the latter.

[25] This is a big problem because they are excluded a priori.

[26] Fellows, 925

[27] It makes sense to me to understand autonomy as being relational. Our sense of self is relational in that we are who we are, in part because of our relations with others (whose identities we play a role in shaping); when we make decisions, we consider others, and others also shape our decisions.

Informed Consent

The prevailing trend in healthcare ethics, at least in Ontario, is to focus on consent as the sole arena of autonomy considerations.[28] It is the duty of healthcare practitioners to get informed consent from their capable patients before providing treatment.[29] The emphasis in bioethics is not so much on what it means to be an autonomous person as it is on being able to act autonomously. If one is capable as that is legally defined, one can make autonomous decisions and vice versa. It is in this way that autonomy and informed consent are generally related.[30] In order to be able to choose to consent or refuse medical treatment, patients must be able to meet the required standards of informed consent, which includes being able to understand the information that is provided, being able to appreciate the reasonably foreseeable consequences of accepting or refusing treatment, and being able to make the choice voluntarily.[31] If patients cannot demonstrate these skills, then they are deemed to be incapable of autonomous decision-making, particularly to a specific medical treatment, at a particular time.[32] Healthcare providers must present appropriate information for their patients to consider. Patients have the right to accept or refuse the treatment.

I have already discussed the limits of understanding autonomy as narrowly defined in terms of rational decision-making. So when we look at informed consent laws, the same concerns are raised. Informed consent laws are meant to ensure that capable people can exercise their right to choose to accept or refuse treatment options presented. This seems like a reasonable plan, albeit only for people who meet the criteria that informed consent requires (these are people who are capable to make autonomous decisions). By and large it excludes many people with dementia from partaking in their own medical decision-making because they are deemed "incapable" and therefore in need of protection.[33]

Also, I have already identified an alternate way to understand autonomy, and that has to do with being "valuers"—that is, holding onto values and interests that are

---

[28] Dodds, 213

[29] Ontario's *Health Care Consent Act, 1996*, S.O. c. 2, s. A., p. 1.4 provides the legal minimum standard that must be met.

[30] It is the critical opinion of some philosophers and ethicists, notably particular feminist theorists and practitioners, that the term "conflated" is a more accurate depiction of the relationship between autonomy and informed consent. For example, see Mackenzie, 5; Dodds, 225. These critics assert that the concept of autonomy has been too narrowly construed in its scope of meaning and application. Proponents of relational autonomy often make this claim.

[31] See Ontario's *Health Care Consent Act, 1996*, S.O. c. 2, s. A., p. 1.4.

[32] In Ontario, autonomous decision-making or capacity is time and domain specific. This means that a person can be considered to be capable of autonomous decision-making in one area, but not necessarily in another, and at one specific time, but not necessarily at another time.

[33] When I refer to the phrase "partaking in medical decision-making," I am referring to a larger view than what the legal construct allows for. I believe many people with dementia can still participate in the process of medical decision-making by having their values and interests inform decision-making.

meaningful to us. This is the only criteria or factor that I believe is relevant in terms of medical decision-making for people with dementia. It serves as an antidote to the traditional view of autonomy as narrowly rationalistic, a view Stephen Post has coined as "hypercognitive."[34]

I further believe that contrary to current practice standards, we ought to "lower the bar," not raise it when it comes to decisions that matter the most for persons.[35] Because social/relational and emotional areas of "intelligence" or "capacity" can remain relatively unscathed in the brains of people with dementia, even into the more severe stages, and because these areas are more associated with values, beliefs, and interests, most people with dementia will be accorded with "autonomy."[36] In any regard, other significant persons in their lives can be actively engaged in assisting them.[37] The idea is that whenever there is uncertainty about what decisions patients with dementia would make, we are morally obliged to try to ascertain from their current behaviors and/or wishes, what values and interests are paramount for them. These should be informative of how decisions on their behalf ought to be made.

---

[34] Stephen G. Post, "Respectare: Moral Respect for the Lives of the Deeply Forgetful," in *Dementia: Mind, Meaning and the Person,* ed. Julian C. Hughes, Stephen J. Louw and Steven R. Sabat (Oxford: Oxford University Press, 2006), 223.

[35] My suggestion is more aligned with the principle of autonomy, which is the standard that the Ontario laws surrounding informed consent are supposed to be applicable to. However, the clinical practice requirement that a capacity threshold be set in (positive) relation to a risk level suggests to me that a protection (best interest or welfare) standard is being used. In fact, it appears to me that, in reality, the practice of informed consent in healthcare organizations is based upon both these principles. While I am addressing informed consent only in relation to autonomy at this point, it will soon become evident that there are many shortcomings that arise when we (mis)understand autonomy to be the trumping principle. For further insights regarding the relationship between informed consent and well-being, see Angus Dawson, "Informed Consent: should we really insist upon it?" *New Review of Bioethics* 1, no. 1(Nov 2003): 64.

[36] See S. Sherwin for further discussion on social and relational competence. Susan Sherwin, "A Relational Approach to Autonomy in Health Care" in *Health Care Ethics in Canada,* ed. F. Baylis, J. Downie, B. Hoffmaster and S. Sherwin (Toronto: Nelson Press, 2nd ed., 2004): 192-208. In addition, Agnieszka Jaworska refers to current findings in neurophysiology and in the neuropathology of Alzheimer's disease to defend the idea that valuing may be quite independent of grasping the narrative of one's life. The disease most severely affects the hippocampus, an area of the brain indispensable for maintaining the sense of one's life as a whole, but not particularly important for the ability to value. Other areas of the brain are mainly responsible for reasoning and decision-making processes, particularly related to feelings and emotions and personal and social matters. A person's ability to value would be more likely to be compromised if these regions were damaged, which happens on an inconsistent basis and in more severe stages. She claims that some but not all of one's former values would likely be lost in the moderate stage. Agnieszka Jaworska, "Respecting the Margins of Agency: Alzheimer's Patients and the Capacity to Value," *Philosophy and Public Affairs* 28, no. 2 (Spring 1999): 121-122.

[37] See Ralf Jox, "Revocation of Advance Directives," In *Advance Directives*, ed. Peter Lack, Nikola Biller-Andorno and Susanne Brauer (New York: Springer, 2014) 74. He asserts that the principle of respect for autonomy requires that every attempt must be made in order to enhance an individual's decision-making capacity.

I begin my ethical analysis of each of the three composite cases by trying to determine if the advance directive meets the criteria of informed consent, laying the groundwork for this more specifically in the first case, pertaining to Mr. Black.[38] In Chap. 2, I also discuss the notion of "autonomy" being more relevant, both conceptually and practically, when understood as pertaining to "having values and interests." I expand on this theme in the case of Mrs. Black, in Chap. 3. The case of Mr. White, in Chap. 4, highlights the difficulties of adhering to a legal model of informed consent. To summarize, the legal model of informed consent is useful in that it helps to ensure that capable people are aware of what they are getting themselves into and that the healthcare providers who have offered the treatment have done due vigilance to disclose all required information and are not coercing their patients. Beyond that I suggest that trying to exclude patients from expressing their desires and wishes if they cannot pass the "capacity" test is misguided. In any case, regardless of the standard being used, a lower threshold ought to be required especially with decisions that matter the most (and might correlate higher with risk) because that is more in line with what autonomy is supposed to be about, that is, allowing people as much as possible to live their lives according to their wishes and values. We should rarely tamper with this. Any involvement should be in the context of "filling the gap" as claimed by Post, to assist those who need help, always with the aim to help them identify and/or express their interests, wishes, and values.[39] Ultimately, medical decision-making ought to be considered in relation to coherence to that which patients value most.

In the following section, we revisit the notion of autonomy, but this time we focus on precedent (or prospective) autonomy. The stage becomes set to begin to critically evaluate what exactly is meant by this term and whether some assumptions generally held about its relationship to the advance directive are in fact true.

Precedent Autonomy

As mentioned, an advance directive is a tool to project our capable treatment wishes into the future time when we may not be deemed legally capable of decision-making. As a tool, an advance directive relies on precedent autonomy. Precedent autonomy refers to the autonomy (ability to make a capable decision according to one's own interests) a person had in the past prior to one's current state as nonautonomous (because not deemed currently to be capable). "This principle recognizes

---

[38] While in Ontario advance directives (the term I use with caveats above, i.e. "wishes") are not conceptualized to meet the standard of informed consent, I explain on page 18 why I undertake this determination.

[39] Post, 229. Also see Olick, 58. He states that "A physician determination of incapacity triggers the authority of the healthcare proxy, but for patients who are interactive, with some capacity for reasoning, this should not categorically exclude them from the decision process…and respect for autonomy encompasses enhancing opportunities for patients to make their own decisions."

that future-oriented actions are integral to the moral life of autonomous persons."[40] In general, precedent autonomy can be understood in contrast to contemporaneous autonomy.[41] Again this gets back to the idea that capable people can make decisions according to their own interests, and others are not to interfere. Because incapable people (legally) cannot make their own decisions and because we as a society believe so strongly in this principle of autonomy, we can honor others' autonomy in the future when they become incapable regarding a specific treatment decision by extending their autonomy from the past (precedent autonomy) into the future time of incapacity.[42,43]

Due to my modification in terms of how to understand autonomy, the dichotomy between precedent and contemporary autonomy collapses. We likely can be valuers all through our lives. However, if we stick with the traditional way of understanding autonomy, there are a number of problems related to precedent autonomy. In Chap. 2, I present the case of Mr. Black and discuss a number of reasons as to why precedent autonomy and contemporary autonomy are not conceptually or morally equivalent. I identify the problems of predictability and irreversibility as two main ones. With reference to the predictability problem, I argue that likely no one can fulfill the legal criteria of consent (at least in Ontario, and probably well beyond this jurisdiction) because nobody can make an informed decision, in part because we cannot know today all the relevant details involved in such a future situation nor can we appreciate all the consequences.[44] In Ontario, at least, informed consent now to a "plan of treatment" in future based on current condition and what is likely to happen in future does exist, such that the capable patient can make choices today knowing the risks and benefits and alternatives; a substitute decision-maker may do so as well. This is not merely a wish, it is a consent that can be acted on, e.g. in the case of a patient with Alzheimer's for whom aspiration pneumonia is likely as the disease becomes severe, and there is a discussion today of what treatment they consent to now, to address that situation in future.

It is almost impossible to pick up an article or book about Alzheimer's dementia without some reference to the notion that there is a split between the "then" person

---

[40] R. Olick, 55

[41] In general use, the term *autonomy* refers to and is interchangeable with the term *contemporaneous autonomy*.

[42] R. Olick, 55. "The oft-recited legal principle grounding advance directive laws is that incompetent patients have the same rights of self-determination as competent patients. Only the means for exercising these important rights should differ."

[43] Ibid, 56. Here Olick states "...the importance of future oriented plans and commitments for how we die (or the legacy we leave our families) survives loss of capacity to appreciate whether those plans and commitments are respected. It still matters whether our wishes, values and decisions near the end of life are honored or disregarded, even if we can no longer know what decisions are taken by our proxy, family and physician."

[44] For a fuller understanding of these issues, see Angus Dawson, "Advance Directives," *General Practice and Ethics*, ed. Christopher Dowrich and Lucy Frith (London: Rutledge, 1999) 130-171; Christopher James Ryan, "Betting your life: an argument against certain advance directives," *Journal of Medical Ethics* 22, no. 6 (1996): 96-99.

(pre-dementia) and the "now" person (post-dementia). The idea of this sort of distinction is incoherent when applied to the notions of autonomy that I suggest. Nonetheless, even when examined within the traditional context as outlined above, I think it is ridiculous to speculate that such a "break" in personhood has occurred. I have already discussed the continued existence of values, which challenges the notion of such a split. Of course the disease of dementia has altered the current patient in significant ways, but it is incoherent to consider that the current patient is "no longer the same person." Values and interests continue on through dementia. Other people can assist in reinforcing these attributes that help sustain the person's identity over time.

Overwhelmingly, advance directives do not meet the criteria for autonomous decision-making in the sense of informed consent. While in the province of Ontario they have not been legally conceptualized as cohering to the standard of informed consent, as they are wishes, not consent, for future treatments, they are premised upon the concept of precedent autonomy and presumed to be morally equivalent to contemporary autonomy, as aforementioned. Informed consent is, after all, the clinical application of the principle of autonomy. Therefore I ask in every chapter if the advance directive meets the standard for informed consent. Directives that are more informed ought to carry more weight. In reality, generally they are not sufficiently informed. This point is well evidenced in the cases of Mr. Black in Chap. 2 and Mrs. Black in Chap. 3. However, the case of Mr. White in Chap. 4 is illuminating in another way. It exemplifies one of the best examples I have to date (of the *rare* occurrence) of an advance directive coming awfully close to meeting the legal standard of informed consent, if not actually meeting it.

The cases I usually provide consultation to often involve substitute decision-makers who act on behalf of incapable persons. In some cases, their role is quite simple, and the steps they are legally required to take (again varying among differing jurisdictions through the Western World) do not usually raise concerns. However, the opposite is at times the case, and many times the issues surrounding substitute decision-making raise a host of ethical challenges that must be faced. The next section provides a brief introduction to set the stage for more robust discussions.

Substitute Decision-Making

When I discuss substitute decision-making in this book, I am referring to the legal obligation that substitute decision-makers (SDMs) are required to undertake according to the jurisdictions they live in.[45] These individuals might have been named in a power of attorney by the respective persons in legal documents or have been legally assigned to act on behalf of others at a time when they were incapable to make their own decisions. Specifically SDMs have a duty to interpret the wishes of the patient

---

[45] For example, see Ontario's *Substitute Decisions Act*, 1992, S.O. c. 30, p. II. Some jurisdictions use the term "proxy" instead of "substitute decision-maker".

for whom treatment is proposed, and on that basis, give or refuse consent to treatment on behalf of persons who are incapable with respect to the treatments at hand.

There are two principles that govern how decisions ought to be made. The default standard is the capable wish principle. If SDMs know of a wish applicable to the circumstances that persons expressed while capable, and after turning a certain age, the SDMs are required to give or refuse consent in harmony with the wishes. If the SDMs do not know of any prior capable wishes, applicable to the circumstances, or if it is not possible to apply the wishes, then the standard to be used is the best interest principle.[46] This principle specifies that current wishes of incapable persons are to be considered, in tandem with what is known about previous values, and taking into account a balancing of current benefits, risks, and consequences. Notwithstanding the challenges inherent within a best interest principle, of which there are many, the most significant moral feature I wish to emphasize is that the current persons' wishes are to be considered. The importance of this principle will be explained in Chap. 3.

In this latter paragraph, I have made several references to "persons" in association with the terms "capable" and "incapable" as well as employing the term "person's current wishes" as distinct from their "prior" wishes. All these terms beg a deeper understanding of "personhood" which I present as the next key concept to be introduced.

Personhood

Many authors debate whether persons with Alzheimer's dementia are the same persons, new persons, or nonpersons, employing an all or nothing view of personhood. In part this is due to the prevalent Western World view that Alzheimer's is a disease that robs persons of their personhood. Partly, the tendency to believe this is due to assigning disproportionate value to rational abilities, rather than appreciating a fuller sense of what constitutes personhood (emotions, spirituality, relationships, etc.).

Arguments advanced by authors who tend to view persons with dementia in such a limited way do not cohere with everyday clinical and practical experiences of caring for patients with diagnoses of Alzheimer's dementia. I cannot recall one instance where the clinician (or family member) stood in front of a patient with dementia and questioned if the "entity" before her was in fact a person. I have heard many comments over a number of years in multiple settings, such as "she is no longer my mother," but clearly the distraught daughter or son is referring to a qualitative change, not a quantitative one. While I do not dispute that the phenomena Alzheimer's and similar forms of dementia can raise philosophically interesting questions about the nature of personhood and diachronic identity, I do not find the converse sufficiently persuasive to make personhood a major focus in my discussion

---

[46] See Ontario's *Health Care Consent Act*, 1996, S.O. c. 2, s. A, p. 59.

of advance directives. In my experience, to question whether patients with dementia are the same persons, new persons, or nonpersons is typically unhelpful.

Now that we have reviewed the main objectives and key concepts that are foundational to this book, it is time to present the cases. As aforementioned in the Preface, in order to protect the privacy and confidentiality of all concerned, the following three case studies are all composites, based upon a variety of common situations I have encountered over many years and in many settings. All of the patients, families, substitute decision-makers, and healthcare practitioners I have portrayed are fictionalized. Any resemblance to known or real persons, living or deceased, is coincidental.

Sources

Atkinson, Jacqueline M. J.M. Advance Directives in Mental Health: Theory, Practice and Ethics. London: Jessica Kingsley Publishers, 2007.

Aquilina, Carmelo and Julian C Hughes. "The Return of the Living Dead: Agency Lost and Found?" In Dementia: Mind, Meaning, and the Person, edited by Julian C. Hughes, Stephen J. Louw and Steven R. Sabat, 143–161. Oxford: Oxford University Press, 2006.

Baylis, F., J. Downie, B. Hoffmaster, and S. Sherwin, eds. Health Care Ethics in Canada. 2nd ed. Toronto: Nelson, 2004.

Beauchamp, T.I., and J.F. Childress. Principles of Biomedical Ethics. New York: Oxford University Press, 2001

Conolly, Ceci. "Obama takes personal approach in AARP speech," The Washington Post, July 29, 2009.

Dawson, Angus. "Informed Consent: Should We Really Insist Upon It?" New Review of Bioethics 1, 1 (November 2003): 59–71.

Dawson, Angus. "Advance Directives." In General Practice and Ethics, edited by Christopher Dowrich and Lucy Fritch, 130–171. London: Rutledge, 1999.

Dodds, Susan. "Choice and Control in Feminist Bioethics." In Relational Autonomy: Feminist Perspectives on Autonomy, Agency and the Social Self, edited by Catriona Mackenzie and Natalie Stoljar, 213–235. Oxford University Press US, 2000.

Dresser, Rebecca. "Dworkin on Dementia: Elegant Theory, Questionable Policy." Hastings Center Report 25, no. 6 (Nov–Dec 1995): 32–38.

Fellows, L.K. "Competency and Consent in Dementia." Journal of the American Geriatrics Society 46, no. 7 (1998): 922–926.

Health Care (Consent) and Care Facility (Admission) Act, R.S.B.C. Health Care (Consent) and Care Facility (Admission) Act, R.S.B.C. 1996, c.

Herskovits, Elizabeth. "Struggling over Subjectivity: Debates about the 'Self' and Alzheimer's Disease." Medical Anthropology Quarterly 9, no. 2 (1995): 146–164.

Jaworska, Agnieszka. "Respecting the Margins of Agency: Alzheimer's Patients and the Capacity to Value." Philosophy and Public Affairs 28, vol. 2 (Spring 1999): 105–138.

Jox, Ralf. "Revocation of Advance Directives." In Advance Directives, edited by P. Lack, N. Biller-Andorno and S. Brauer. New York: Springer Press, 2014.

Olick, Robert S. "On the Scope and Limits of Advance Directives and Prospective Autonomy." In Advance Directives, edited by P. Lack, N. Biller-Andorno and S. Brauer. New York: Springer Press, 2014.

Post, Stephen G. "Respectare: Moral Respect for the Lives of the Deeply Forgetful." In Dementia: Mind, Meaning, and the Person, edited by Julian C. Hughes, Stephen J. Louw and Steven R. Sabat, 223–234. Oxford: Oxford University Press, 2006.

Sabat, Steven R. "Capacity for Decision-Making in Alzheimer's Disease: Selfhood, Positioning and Semiotic People." Australian and New Zealand Journal of Psychiatry 39, no. 11–12 (November 2005): 1030–1035.

Sailors, Pam R. "Autonomy, Benevolence, and Alzheimer's Disease." Cambridge Quarterly of Healthcare Ethics 10 (2001): 184–193.

Seymour, Jane and Horne, Gillian. "Advance Care Planning for the end of life: an overview" in Advance Care Planning in End of Life Care, edited by K. Thomas and B. Lobo, 18. Oxford: Oxford University Press, 2011.

Sherwin, Susan. "A Relational Approach to Autonomy in Health Care." 2nd ed. In Health Care Ethics in Canada, edited by F. Baylis, J. Downie, B. Hoffmaster and S. Sherwin, 192–208. Toronto: Nelson Press, 2004.

Simon, Alfred. "Historical Review of Advance Directives. In Advance Directives, edited by P. Lack, N. Biller-Andorno and S. Brauer, 3–16. New York: Springer Press, 2014.

Chapter 2
Mr. Black

I will begin with a case that one might perceive as quite straightforward and unproblematic, with the hope of shedding light on why some cases are perceived to be more problematic and nuanced than others.

Mr. Black

Five years ago, at the age of 75, Mr. Black, a retired family law lawyer and mediator, married and a father of three adult children, and grandfather to seven, began to experience short-term memory lapses explained by his physician as due to normal aging. As an attorney, he knew something about the merit of advance directives. Frightened by the future prospect of a potential full-blown dementia (he had witnessed his best friend's physical and mental demise due to dementia), he spent a few days considering what he should write in his own advance directive. He had been primed by his lawyer to think about his current values and interests and to ensure he took them into consideration when he wrote his advance directive. Mr. Black completed the advance directive form his lawyer gave him, stating that if he could no longer enjoy the kinds of activities he found pleasurable, such as bird watching and hiking with his wife, walking his two poodles, dining at fine restaurants, or engaging in debates with his adult children and grandchildren, he would wish to receive no treatment except pain treatment, if diagnosed with an incurable disease. He stated that living under those conditions would be unbearable for him.

Currently, Mr. Black is an 80-year-old gentleman with moderate to severe stage Alzheimer's dementia. He is a patient in a hospital rehabilitation unit, having recently sustained a hip fracture from falling out of his bed in a long-term care residence where he has been living for the past 3 years. In addition to the usual medical care offered in his unit, he has been receiving around-the-clock personal attendant care—privately hired—for all his hygiene and daily living requirements. Bedridden, except for occupational therapy treatment sessions, he spends most of the day

M. Sokolowski, *Dementia and the Advance Directive*,
https://doi.org/10.1007/978-3-319-72083-8_2

sleeping. He is receiving pain medicine that seems to alleviate most of his discomfort, although when awake he often moans and tries to shift his body, appearing uncomfortable and somewhat agitated. He does not speak, has trouble swallowing, and is fed pureed foods. His physician is concerned about Mr. Black's decreasing ability to swallow, having treated two recent bouts of pneumonia most likely the result of food aspiration due to Mr. Black's impaired swallow reflex. A short while ago, the doctor informed the family that they will need to consider the option of having a feeding tube inserted, since Mr. Black is unable to intake enough nutrition to maintain his daily nutritional needs.

Mr. Black often fleetingly fastens his gaze on his family members, particularly on his wife, sister, and youngest granddaughter, when they are present, but remains mainly expressionless. When asked simple questions requiring a "yes" or "no" response, there is no discernible indication that he understands nor is he able to respond in a meaningful way. These perceptions are shared by Mr. Black's family, respective staff members, and hired attendants. His emotional responses appear muted, probably somewhat due to his pain medication. His wife in particular is mournful about what she describes as "the gradual loss and disappearance of my husband" over time. At the same time, she thoughtfully reflects that she has never stopped loving him and "sees occasional glimpses of the person he was." Mrs. Black often refers to the past when he was "a highly intelligent and successful lawyer" and misses the numerous activities they shared together. She speaks of "getting used to his demise" over the past 3 years and says that she is comforted by sitting near him and holding his hand, gently soothing him when he gets restless. His children share a sense of relief that their father seems to have moved from the "I remember that I often forget" stage of earlier Alzheimer's dementia to what they deem to be his current "I forget that I forget" later stage, since now his agitation seems to also be decreased. "He no longer seems to be aware of losing himself" is how they put it.

Two weeks later, Mr. Black is diagnosed with another bout of severe pneumonia. The doctor explains that antibiotics might again be curative. However, he feels that Mr. Black is at a high risk for recurrent aspirations resulting from oral feedings and possible death as a result. He asks Mr. Black if he would want a feeding tube, though he (correctly) expects him to be incapable of responding. The doctor calls in the interdisciplinary team and family to discuss the option of a feeding tube.

The doctor reviews the potential benefits, risks, and consequences. In particular, he stresses the potential adverse consequences of having a feeding tube in great detail. These possible consequences include a stomach rupture, with resultant bleeding, recurrent aspirations, heart failure, as well as infection at the insertion site. The designated legal attorney for personal care is Mrs. Black. She notifies the team that her husband has an advance directive and she produces a copy of it. It stipulates what his wishes would be at a later point in time, if incapable to express himself. The doctor reads the advance directive aloud. There is unanimous agreement that the situation Mr. Black described in his advance directive seems to match the current situation. Of greater relevance is the fact that Mrs. Black must interpret his wishes, as she is the one legally required to do so. Since her husband is not able to express capable wishes at this time, nor has he been able to do so for a long time, the advance directive is referred to, as it represents his most recent capable wishes. In line with what he had written, everyone is in agreement that he should not receive any treatment for his pneumonia, with the understanding that his death will likely occur in a few days. With the consent of his substitute decision-maker, he will be provided with comfort measures only, including continued pain medication. Mr. Black dies in his sleep 4 days later with his family at his bedside. Professional team members and family members feel that they have done the "right thing" by acting in accordance with his wishes as captured in the advance directive (in this case, a power of attorney), and as interpreted by his substitute decision-maker.

Discussion and Analyses

Each case is, of course, unique. There are individual and group dynamics among and between family and team members, further influenced by the culture, beliefs, and policies of the organization that shape the kind of interactions and ethics-related decisions that are made at any one time. Analyses of such a complex system can never be complete or definitively conclusive. Nonetheless, there are some key issues that I will discuss at this point in order to highlight the idiosyncratic nature of each case and to demonstrate how a change in reaction of even one member of the team or family could influence how advance directives are interpreted and responded to.

Why Did This Case Present Little, If Any, Moral Distress or Ethical Concern?

(a) There were shared perception and agreement among all staff and family members about all major issues raised. For instance, everyone agreed that Mr. Black was unable to express any capable wishes with regard to acceptance or refusal of a feeding tube. Moreover, everyone also agreed that the situation Mr. Black faced now matched the conditions he had addressed in his advance directive. He could no longer enjoy the social and recreational activities he had in the past, he could not interact in a meaningful way with his children, and he had an incurable dementia with associated cognitive and physical deterioration. Mr. Black's mood seemed to range from appearing dull or lifeless to agitated and irritable. While the family felt that more recently he was less frustrated, possibly because he was no longer aware of having a dementia, they did view him to be generally unhappy. In the scenario I have created here, he had explicitly stated that living in this way would be unbearable for him. This mood seemed to match what he spoke of in his directive: the prospect of his life becoming more unbearable. He did develop an illness, namely, pneumonia, requiring treatment to keep him alive, and he was clear he did not wish treatment in the face of having an incurable disease (Alzheimer's). Nobody voiced any difficulties with interpreting the wishes set out in his advance directive and applying it to the current situation.

While it is up to the SDM to interpret the wishes, the team members intrerpretations happened to match those of the SDM, resulting in absence of moral distress.

I think the situation might have proved to be much more challenging in a case where a family believed the patient was currently happy most of the time. The difference this might have made, in terms of wanting to override his advance directive, is shown in the Chap. 3 case scenario. It is easy to equate expressions of happiness with good quality of life, and it is not hard to imagine how difficult it can be to know that either no treatment will be offered or treatment will be terminated, in accordance with the advance directive.[1] Often, there is someone who will argue that the advance directive should not be honored because, if the patient could express his wishes today, he would opt for treatment to try to extend his life.[2] Intuitively, following the directive just does not seem like the "right" thing to do. We will return to this sort of difficult situation in Chap. 3.

(b) Another reason that this case presented so few ethical challenges was because nobody viewed Mr. Black as a completely different or new person. Even though the family felt Mr. Black's "old self was lost," sometimes they caught glimpses of "who he used to be." I mention this now because believing that the patient is so changed that he is no longer the same person as the one who wrote the advance directive leads some to conclude that the directive should no longer apply, given that person A cannot bind a different person, person B, to person A's former or present wishes.

(c) Mr. Black's decline was gradual, and there was a sense that the family got used to his decline over time. They seemed more emotionally prepared to deal with his loss and were "ready" to let him go.

The reactions of families often have a big impact on what ethical issues arise and how they are resolved. For example, I have witnessed family members becoming extremely distressed in the face of potential loss of loved ones and, in moments of desperation and panic, asking to override their advance directives in order to prolong the lives of their loved ones. Especially in situations where death is imminent, if treatments are not attempted, as when someone is choking and an advance directive calls for no intervention, it is easy to understand how a substitute decision-maker would order treatments to be initiated, despite knowing that their loved ones have requested otherwise, and that their role is not to advance their own wishes but to interpret the patient's. Sometimes family

---

[1] On the other hand, even though Mr. Black appeared to be quite unhappy, we cannot be sure that he would not have wanted to have his life extended. Perhaps, even in his current state, he had found his life to have new meaning.

[2] While this may be the most frequently cited argument I encounter, there are other reasons given as well, which will be identified in the next chapter.

members or substitute decision-makers demand that either emergency interventions occur immediately or that 911 be called if the staff are unwilling to intervene or are not equipped to do so because of medical limitations or policies.

When family members of substitute decision-makers attempt to override advance directives in such circumstances, often a number of difficult ethical challenges arise, mainly pertaining to moral distress. Staff may feel they are colluding in doing harm to patients if they "send them out" or may be concerned about potential physical harm to the patients through aggressive treatment, for example, breaking ribs when CPR is applied. Many staff members are worried that patients may survive, but will do so at the cost of ending up in even more compromised positions than before. Ultimately, they are deeply concerned about issues of breach of trust between them and the family members. This is why I recommend that, whenever possible, staff should explain to family members that a sudden state of panic, with associated desires to provide all resuscitation techniques to their loved ones, is a likely and understandable reaction. To be able to override this crisis reaction requires that staff be proactive and spend sufficient time preparing and supporting family members and substitute decision-makers in advance, so that they do not succumb to crisis mode emotional decisions. And yet, even in the face of compelling advance directives to withhold treatment, when the family members witnessed what might have signaled the patients' dying last breaths, some will insist on calling for an ambulance to take their loved ones to an acute care unit or emergency center.[3]

It is a moment of panic, in the moment of crisis. Often, these patients die in the ambulance or in the emergency department. The receiving hospitals feel frustrated that patients who have advance directives requesting no such intervention are sent to them, often taking issue with the originating healthcare organizations that sent on the patients. The same thing happens at the receiving facilities. The medical staff members do not feel they should provide treatment and argue that they are "doing harm" to the patients. The substitute decision-makers who succeed in getting the treatment they want for the patients often witness resuscitation measures far more traumatic than they had envisioned, including their frail elderly charges left with broken ribs and often in a much more disabled state than before.

In that sort of situation, if a substitute decision-maker argues that the patient's directive is for some reason or another not applicable in the current situation (e.g., if the SDM says that the patient had a change of mind later and did not update the written document), who is there in the emergency situation to challenge or

---

[3] Thiel discusses how difficult it can be for the proxy to "do nothing when *doing* is so important." Marie-Jo Thiel, "Personal Capacity to Anticipate Future Illness and Treatment Preferences," *Advance Directives,* ed. Peter Lack, Nikola Biller-Andorno and Susanne Brauer (New York: Springer, 2014); 21.

disqualify these assertions?[4] Different jurisdictions within countries may have legal venues available to access in such situations, but my belief is that not many practitioners want to end up in an adversarial position in a court of law arguing against keeping patients alive, even if they believe this is what their patients stated in the advance directive. How can staff be sure that their patients did not have a change of mind later that was expressed to the SDM? At times, the sending units in such cases will tell the respective families, if their patients survive, that they will not readmit the patients, unless the substitute decision-makers are willing to adhere to the patients' most recently expressed capable wishes. Usually, once these crises have blown over, the teams and families can reflect together on what happened and agree on plans for the future that do not depart from the previous wishes of the capable patients. Agreement is usually reached when the discussions are open, feelings and values are made transparent, and trust is established.

Unfortunately, however, it is often those patients whose wishes (not to receive treatment) have been violated who end up paying the biggest price. Not only is their will not respected, but both their dignity and their bodies are violated by having aggressive treatment measures applied, rendering them more vulnerable, more disabled, and more than ever needing to be able to trust their loved ones.

Medical decision-making involves not only patients, family members, and physicians in charge but also the entire multidisciplinary teams, including social workers, nursing professionals, dieticians, occupational therapists, physiotherapists, recreation therapists, speech therapists, and others as required, including ethicists, chaplains, and music therapists. There is a belief that bringing staff together from different professional backgrounds adds richness and depth to the decision-making process. Because of the divergent perspectives that these staff bring, sometimes there can be important differences in how to interpret the medical situations, the patients' comfort levels, and other factors that are considered in decision-making. For example, sometimes a team member who is working very closely with a patient over a very long period of time learns to interpret the patient's body language and gestures in such a way as to know what the patient is asking for or its meaning to convey. While others might claim that the patient is not capable to make a particular decision, this particular team member might argue that the patient is capable to some degree and that the patient's gestures should be seriously considered. Whatever we say about the epistemology of such judgments, it is clear that the staff are professionally well-motivated. Nonetheless, conflicting interpretations of patients and their treatments can result in any health care setting.

---

[4] I recall a case where all five adult children strongly argued that their father's very extensive, highly descriptive advance directive should not be honored because they all knew he wrote it when very depressed and likely incapable, and "only wrote it out of a fit of intense sadness." Their father recovered from his depression a few weeks later and "went on his usual merry way" and, his children alleged, never even remembered he had written it. They forcefully argued it was "not our father" who wrote it then, as he was "under the spell of a broken heart." The staff members were unwilling to challenge the family members who were the substitute decision-makers in this case. Some felt that the children's argument was a potentially justifiable one. Perhaps he indeed was not capable when he wrote it.

In addition, there may be different views about how to measure capacity: how high or low to set the bar and how to interpret or assess suffering. Consider a situation where the healthcare team is attempting to devise a medical plan of care based predominantly on pain control. Some members perceive the patient to be experiencing severe suffering, some see it as moderate, and some consider it mild. I attribute these variances to a variety of factors, including different observation times, applying different standards to the measurement of suffering, and also interpretation differences. The staff member who perceived the patient to be suffering the least was someone who mainly worked in a trauma unit where she was often exposed to acute and severe suffering. Being temporarily assigned to cover a chronic care long-term unit where the patient was often seen moaning and grimacing, she brought with her, so to speak, her previous long-established frame of reference. She did not have the benefit that other staff had of getting to know this patient over a longer period of time. Nonetheless, even among staff members who did know the patient for about the same time period and observed her at the same time, ratings differed significantly. It is obvious that there is a great deal of subjectivity involved, influenced by professional practice experience, attitudes, and values about pain and suffering, cultural contexts, and religious beliefs.

So Whose View Is "Right?"

We can now see how subjective experiences influence the opinions of team members and how these differences, in turn, could be communicated to other staff and family members. The case of Mr. White, discussed in Chap. 4, will demonstrate these issues more starkly. These kinds of differences do not just arise among healthcare team members. They are just as commonly found between family members as well. While we might be talking about objective medical diagnoses, the attitudes toward these diseases, opinions about prognosis, values, and beliefs of respective stakeholders are all largely subjective. I have already made reference to what has been called the "social construction" of disease: the meanings that particular societies place on particular diseases or diagnoses. Remember that the usual description of dementia in North America is that it is a disease that robs the person of her "self" and is generally considered to be a living nightmare. The interpretations we assign to the condition play a huge role in how attitudes and beliefs about its diagnosis, prognosis, and treatment options are experienced, communicated, and shaped.

The general feeling on the part of Mr. Black's family and team members was that they were all very satisfied with how well it worked to have an advance directive, a written expression of him wishes. Moral distress was kept to an extreme minimum, and they all felt good about being able to honor Mr. Black's wishes. They also expressed positive sentiments with regard to the ease with which they were able to work together, keeping the interests of Mr. Black in the foreground. There was no doubt that they felt this to be an example of a case that "worked exceptionally well" and much of the credit went to the foresight of Mr. Black for creating his advance directive in the first place.

Mrs. Black, her children, and the team believed they were complying with the advance directive, and in the absence of any challenges to the contrary, there would be no impetus to think otherwise. Sometimes, there is the perception that the advance directive is not applicable to the current circumstances and thus should not be followed. However, this was not the case in this situation. Nobody overtly challenged their own or anyone else's opinions and perceptions. In particular, nobody pressed the issue that perhaps Mr. Black had so significantly changed during this period of his life as a dementia patient that it might be ludicrous to believe that his current situation matched the one he identified in his advance directive. Perhaps one or more stakeholders held an opposing thought, but if so, they chose to remain silent.

Recall that recently, prior to the issue of a feeding tube being raised, Mr. Black had suffered two bouts of pneumonia and received antibiotic treatment for each of them. He was deemed incapable to make an informed decision regarding treatment wishes at these times and his SDM consented on his behalf to him being treated during both previous occasions. Mrs. Black had not notified the team of the existence of his advance directive during those times. She may have felt confident that she was following his wishes and nobody questioned her decision to consent to her husband receiving antibiotics. Her interpretation may have included the belief that he wished treatments that might be curative, such as antibiotics for pneumonia. And/or, her intention for consenting to antibiotics may have been for pain reduction. However, one of the team members, upon learning about the existence of the advance directive, questioned if Mr. Black should have previously received antibiotics given he had an incurable disease, namely Alzheimer's, and that according to his interpretation of the advance directive, it was irrelevant if he happened to have a parallel curable disease. However, he did also wonder if the receipt of antibiotics was justifiable due to potential effects of pain control. Similar questions were raised by the same team member with regard to whether or not Mr. Black should have received rehabilitation treatment after he sustained a hip fracture. Nonetheless, how written wishes are interpreted and applied lie with the SDM, and can create some moral struggles for team members.

Let us imagine perhaps that Mrs. Black did believe that consenting to antibiotics previously, and hip treatment was contrary to her husband's advance directive wishs. Maybe she was not emotionally ready to allow him to die at that particular time and thus withheld the existence of his advance directive. Again, hypothetically, if team members were made previously aware of the advance directive they may have also been in agreement of trying to cure his pneumonia or at least to prolong his life. So it may not be unusual for staff members to be in support of trying some intervention, at least once, with SDM consent. Obviously, personal values and beliefs influence how one will act. Those working in a chronic care unit become accustomed to treating and caring for patients who are often very ill. This may result in heightened feelings of protection for these patients, which may result in a desire to prolong their lives. Particularly with patients who seem lonely and do not have many family members or friends visiting, it is easy for staff to develop very caring feelings toward them, perhaps not unlike loving family members. Also, patients may be living in a specific unit or facility for a number of years, so it is not unlikely that benevolent feelings develop. And it is also easy to see how loving family members might "overlook" the fact that there is an advance directive, as they themselves are not ready for their beloved to die.[5] Also, being an ethicist having worked in a variety of healthcare facilities and nursing homes, my experience is that while many do have a formal process in place that easily tracks the existence of advance directives and specific locations where they can be accessed in a hurry, if necessary, some systems are more efficient than others. Of note is that in this case the SDM likely understood the legal mandate and role expectations of the SDM. From my experience across many settings, I can confidently say, sometimes there is an erroneous belief in existence that substitute decision-makers are supposed to replace the decisions of (now incapable) patients with their own. In other words, they think they are to make decisions according to their own wishes, beliefs, and values. This misconception unfortunately applies not only to family members and friends who are substitute decision-makers, but also, albeit rarely to some staff members as well (acknowledging, of course, that staff can never assume the role of substitute decision-maker).[6] This speaks to the importance of the role of education in informing patients, family members, substitute decision-makers, and staff of the legal role of the SDM. Some organizations are better at doing this than are others.

It is very tempting to think that we can project our own wishes about medical treatment into a future time when we will no longer be able to express capable wishes. But this view presupposes many substantial conditions. One challenge is that interpretation of the advance directive is subjective. As the hypothetical elements in this case study discussed in this chapter demonstrates, the everyday practice does not always square with the theory. Substitute decision-makers do not always comply with the advance directives, one reasons being that they may lack full information. This problem might be corrected through proper education, as indicated above; though even with full understanding, there are situations where advance directives are not followed. As I just mentioned, SDMs might also have misconceptions about the roles and mandates of substitute decision-making and how advance directives figure into medical decision-making. To be fair, there is no "crash course" available to them; and it falls on staff to lay out, often at a time of healthcare crisis, the SDM's roles and responsibilities.

---

[5] Robert Olick, "On the Scope and Limits of Advance Directives and Prospective Autonomy," Advance Directives, ed. Peter Lack, Nikola Biller-Andorno and Susanne Brauer (New York: Springer, 2014) 66.

[6] In Chap. 4, I will revisit the topic of substitute decision-making in greater detail.

Further Issues with Mr. Black's Case

(a) The legal requirements for informed consent are a minimum standard.[7]

    The legal requirements for informed consent to treatment include being able to understand the information that is provided, including risks and benefits, being provided the alternatives, being able to appreciate the consequences of accepting or refusing the medical treatment, and being able to make choices voluntarily. This is quite different than the capacity to write an advance directive (i.e., a power of attorney for personal care under Ontario's *Substitute Decisions Act*, which does not necessitate provision of risks and benefits and alternatives). In addition, even a prima facie straightforward case like Mr. Black's shows us that these requirements are not equal to the subtleties and complexities of situations in which consent becomes an issue. I propose augmenting the requirements in the following way: a person writing an advance directive must also understand and appreciate the risks and benefits of having an advance directive versus not having one. This, in turn, would require being informed about other legal standards and procedures that come into play in the absence of an advance directive. We are not only talking about understanding the information regarding treatment wishes and appreciating their consequences. We also need to understand the information pertinent to an advance directive in general, including one's own specifically.[8] Each of these elements, crucial to making an informed decision about making an advance directive, is both practically and conceptually fraught with problems, yet I am unaware whether practical or conceptual clarification is indeed explained for people contemplating an advance directive. As a professional working in the field, I think it seriously undermines the moral (and possibly legal) authority of advance directives if the consequences of having one (versus not having one) are not understood.

    Did Mr. Black meet the requirements of informed consent when he wrote his advance directive? Probably not, probably, nobody could. To have done so would mean that he understood he could become incapacitated to the point where he would be unable to experience the pleasures he enjoyed in interacting with his spouse and adult children. There is no definition provided in Ontario's *Health Care Consent Act* of the term "understand," but generally it seems to

---

[7] The attainment of "fully" informed consent is an ideal that cannot be achieved, but nonetheless should be strived for. As the late Benjamin Freeman said, "There is no end to 'fully informing' patients." See Benjamin Freedman, "Chapter 6: Informed Consent and the Competent Patient," in *Readings in Biomedical Ethics: a Canadian Focus,* 2nd ed., edited by Eike-Henner W. Kluge (Scarborough: Prentice Hall, 1999): 71. We should, I add, try to ensure *everyone* is "sufficiently informed" though there are of course differing opinions on what exactly that means.

[8] For example, in some Canadian provinces, including Ontario, a substitute decision-maker is the person responsible for applying/interpreting the wishes of the patient, not the physician.

mean having the rational ability to grasp the concepts involved.[9] In theory, Mr. Black would need to be able to understand the various scenarios. He would also need to be able to "appreciate" the consequences of what he was requesting. Again, there is no definition of "appreciation" in the relevant legislation in Ontario. The usual understanding of "appreciation" is that one must be able to understand what it means for a specific scenario to be applied to oneself. Sometimes it is termed *emotional understanding*.

So, at the time he is writing his advance directive, Mr. Black needs to be able to imagine himself as incapacitated and quite "otherwise" to how he is currently. Furthermore, he needs to be able to predict how he will experience himself in the context of his life as someone incapacitated. The challenging, perhaps impossible, task he faces is to make an informed decision *now*—in the context of being capable and having the life he has now, the values, beliefs, wishes, and dreams as applicable to him currently—about his *future* self in a very different context as a very ill patient with dementia. Mr. Black has to be able to imagine what that future life would be like for him and what his subjective experience of it would be, including what it would "feel like" for him. And on the basis of this imagining, he also has to make predictions *now* about what kind of medical treatment he would *subsequently* want to refuse or accept.[10]

An advance directive written with contemplation of a dementia diagnosis in the future requires vastly greater imaginative prowess than do most other kinds of decisions that we tend to make. I doubt we are capable of the task. To complicate matters further, I have rarely heard of any advance directive that was written with any input from a medical practitioner in this context. In order to understand the information pertaining to refusal or acceptance of any medical treatment, let alone be able to appreciate the consequences, there would need to be relevant and sufficient medical information given to the person to ponder about dementia. *I think this is rarely done comprehensively, if at all.*

However, if we assume for the moment that Mr. Black would in fact receive *some* relevant medical information about a future scenario, it is probable that he would be able to understand it, although the amount of information would always be incomplete because nobody could anticipate the fullness of every possible scenario. We cannot know now what advances in medical research and technology will be available in the future. Furthermore, I think that regardless of how imaginative Mr. Black's mind might be, being able to appreciate himself as being quite different than he is currently is a very tall order. Of course I cannot prove

---

[9] However, there is a requirement that the treatment provider who is requesting consent describe the treatment in ways that a *reasonable* person would be able to understand (emphasis added). I am not sure at all I would be able to even begin to know how to define a "reasonable" person for this context, but we will leave that problem alone for the moment until I address it in Chap. 3.

[10] Thiel, 22, 24. She stresses that the uncertainties related to anticipation can be so great when one is healthy and stating preferences for (non)treatment of future hypothetical conditions that perhaps these directives ought not to be honored as they cannot be sufficiently informed. She further states that it is because of such uncertainties that France, for example, limits the period of validity of advance directives and/or allows room for their interpretation.

this. However, I think we have evidence in general to the contrary, mainly owing to the fact that our beliefs and values can indeed shift in unforeseen and surprising ways when we experience significant life changes. Research demonstrates that we are in fact poor predictors of what will matter to us and what wishes and values we will hold dear in such a situation.[11] Reliably exercising this personal and moral imagination would require answering some clearly vexing questions. What if I am so different in the future that I no longer hold the same values or wishes? What if I change my mind and cannot capably express this change of mind? What if I am able to express myself, but others think I am incapable so they do not place much value on what I am saying? Will I be a stranger to my past self?

The difficulty in answering these questions about the future is underscored by the reasonable suspicion that we do not always know ourselves so well even in the present. Currently, as long as we are considered to be capable, we are allowed to change our minds, about most things anyway. If we are considered incapable in the future, we will not be allowed to do so, at least from a legal point of view. If these concerns, which constitute some of the relevant consequences of having an advance directive, are not *considered* by us, let alone *appreciated*, how could it be argued that there was informed consent (or even a situation of being sufficiently informed)? I doubt that most people in the midst of writing an advance directive are even alerted to the existence of these kinds of limitations.

Furthermore, we cannot know if the level of appreciation that Mr. Black experienced met suitable standards because we do not have any objective criteria of measurement (recall that the Ontario's *Health Care Consent Act* does not provide a definition of "appreciation"). This leaves us to glean the extent of Mr. Black's grasp of his advance directive from fragmentary and indirect evidence. Mr. Black did witness the demise of a loved one in a similar condition. Perhaps he had some personal experience with capable issues in his own past. We can hardly guess with any confidence. These kinds of experiences might add some weight to an "appreciation score" so to speak, though perhaps only to the "understanding" part. In addition to the problem of not knowing how to measure these "abilities" of imagination and prediction, there is, as mentioned, the additional problem of now knowing what criteria the "assessor" is using or if there even is such a person who is guiding the author of the directive. Perhaps the culture of dementia will in the future itself have changed significantly as well, with people not fearing the disease as much. Who knows? Certainly we do not know this currently. Advance directives are fraught with such unknowns, rendering the question of informed consent, or, even of being sufficiently informed, a deeply problematic one.

When we are of sound enough mind to consider future decision-making scenarios, at a time when we are no longer able to express a competent treatment decision, we are deeply influenced not only by what we see when we observe

---

[11] Angus Dawson, "Advance Directives," *General Practice and Ethics*, ed. Christopher Dowrich and Lucy Frith (London: Rutledge, 1999) 130–171; Christopher James Ryan, "Betting your life: an argument against certain advance directives," *Journal of Medical Ethics* 22, no. 6 (1996): 96–99

people with dementia but by how our society depicts the experience and meaning of such an illness. There already exist important differences in the way different sociocultural groups view and respond to Alzheimer's disease.[12]

Currently the most dominant North American understanding of the meaning of Alzheimer's disease is that it is a neurological illness entailing "loss of personhood" or self, largely due to memory impairment. This definition is intertwined with other notions mentioned in Chap. 1 such as diminished capable, questionable ability to consent to medical treatments, and negative personality changes. If Mr. Black entertains thoughts about how his life might be should he develop Alzheimer's dementia, he will likely view that disease in the negative light in which it is usually depicted. Will he also entertain thoughts that the current stereotypes of this disease might change over time? Will Mr. Black consider that by the time he could be diagnosed, he might consider this diagnosis less or more ghastly than he does now?

When Mr. Black wrote his advance directive, who guided him? Aside from some minimal advice from his lawyer, who assumed that because of Mr. Black's legal background he was already somewhat informed about advance directives, let's assume Mr. Black received no professional advice or support to complete his advance directive. We might assume that the lawyer who signed off for Mr. Black was satisfied, but we do not know if he provided Mr. Black with even the minimum standard of information required (whatever that might be) or a thoughtful enough *process* to ensure that Mr. Black could satisfy the requirements of an autonomous and informed decision. And yet, astonishingly, Mr. Black's efforts went well beyond what is actually required for an advance directive. An advance directive does not necessarily require that a lawyer support or inform the process.[13] Mr. Black could have hurriedly scribbled a few lines on an airplane dinner napkin. Or, he may have downloaded a directive from the Internet and filled it out hurriedly, perhaps after downing a few too many beers, and nobody would necessarily have known the difference.

Mr. Black was a practicing lawyer for many years, so chances are he was aware of the legal status and benefits and limitations of an advance directive in general, probably more so than the average person would be. Nonetheless, we do not know if Mr. Black seriously considered all the risks and benefits of having an advance directive and was really able to appreciate them. As well, being a lawyer likely has no bearing on how skilled he might be in the areas of imagination and prediction. In fact, it is possible that as a lawyer who appreciates intellectual debates, it might have been harder for him to imagine himself as cognitively incapacitated. As well, there was no known concern about his capable level at the time of having written his advance directive. Mr. Black's immediate family believed that his advance directive was well thought out and not an

---

[12] See M.B. Holstein, "Ethics and Alzheimer's disease: widening the lens," *Journal of Clinical Ethics* 9, no. 1 (1998): 13–22.

[13] There is no such legal requirement in Ontario when executing a power of attorney for property or for personal care, but other jurisdictions may have different legal requirements.

impulsive undertaking, which in their minds gave them greater confidence in believing it represented "who he was" and "what he really wanted." At no point did any team or family member ever raise any concerns or questions about the legitimacy of his advance directive. The integrity of his advance directive seemed to be beyond question for them. This is not in the least bit unusual. Rarely does anyone raise this kind of question.[14,15] Having an advance directive is still a fairly rare event, and often the initial response is to be grateful that one even exists. Usually, there is no event that would trigger someone suggesting such a review of the advance directive's legitimacy. The general attitude toward advance directives in the medical care professions seems to be mainly positive, and the attention that has been paid to any cautionary tales varies. I am not sure that most people would think to question their usefulness. The preparation process of an advance directive can be severely lacking, and yet, the directive may be assumed by those charged with applying it to be valid "on its face".

It should be obvious by now that there are reasons to doubt the soundness of the very notion of an advance directive. Let us say that Mr. Black knew enough to consider that sometimes people with dementia might have a change of heart or might no longer perceive Alzheimer's to be such a terrible thing. In fact, suppose that he himself had witnessed some people in this exact situation. Or, let us assume that he knew that his predictive ability was somewhat faulty. Would this knowledge add credibility to his advance directive? Potentially it could, particularly if he were to cite this concern and suggest how the substitute decision-maker might respond to any caution specifically noted in his directive.

Lurking in the background of these specific issues with Mr. Black is a crucial and more general question:

(b) Are the decisions we make in the form of an advance directive (based on precedent autonomy) in the event of future "incapacity" significantly different from the more usual decisions we make?

The short answer is yes.

One difference has to do with the amount of time that elapses between when the decision is made and when it is to be carried out. The other has to do with the degenerative nature of dementia and the subsequent changes that occur in the person. The specific problems that arise are generally associated with one or both of these factors.

I think it is fair to assume that as more time goes by, there may be more opportunities for unanticipated events to intrude. In the case of the advance directive, once an individual is incapacitated and can no longer change these instructions, it could become increasingly misrepresentative and misleading.

---

[14] We will discover, however, an exception to this rule when it comes to the case of Mr. White in Chap. 4.

[15] Thiels, 22. In Austria it is required that one or two witnesses are appointed in order to "bind" the directive and to increase the chances of a free and informed expression of patient wishes, as well as to clarify wishes and expectations.

For example, perhaps Mr. Black might even enjoy the kinds of experiences he could have while having a disease of dementia. Likely, he did not know or appreciate that social/emotional memories might linger into even the more advanced stages of dementia and that he would be perceived to be reaping great rewards from having his wife sit at his bedside daily. Perhaps, shortly after his last pneumonia, there would be a cure for dementia. In Mr. Black's case, however, his advance directive was not written decades before, so chances are it was more relevant than if it had been written years before.[16]

In summary, then, there are two major problems with the responsible implementation of advance directives: irreversibility of the articulated wish and predictive difficulties.

Plausibly, it would be prudent to assume that irreversible decisions regarding one's wishes ought to be made with particular certainty. But how can we increase certainty given that, by definition, the kind of future circumstances relevant to advance directives remain largely unknown, unpredictable, and impossible to appreciate? As noted, there is the possibility in Ontario of a patient signing a consent to a plan of treatment under the *Health Care Consent Act*, based on current diagnosis and what is likely to occur in future. That is not merely a wish, it is a consent that can be relied on directly by the healthcare provider; and it may be given by an SDM.

Of course, many types of decisions that we make also involve imagining ourselves to be in situations not easily imaginable and are also made without a great deal of certainty. The decision to become parents is a prime example. It is not uncommon for new parents to claim that no amount of information or imagination sufficed as ample preparation. "You have to experience it to know it" is a sentiment expressed fairly regularly by new parents. As already stated, research supports the view that we are poor predictors of how we will experience ourselves in radically different situations. Perhaps our values might radically change and, so too, our ideas about what constitutes a good life. Many able-bodied persons imagine they would never want to live if paralyzed and wheelchair bound. Yet, when faced with that situation, many do not wish to have their lives ended. Not all adjust well, but many report that their quality of life is at least satisfactory.

Indeed, there are similarities between advance directive decisions and the more common types of everyday decisions. However, an advance directive,

---

[16] However, while the increasing passage of time does allow for more unanticipated events to occur, there could be examples where the passage of more time could work to one's benefit. For example, because we cannot predict how someone with dementia might respond, it is equally possible that someone might respond in a way that coheres with what was anticipated in the advance directive. So, in this context passage of time would not be the significant factor, given the randomness of chance. In general, however, people do not radically transform themselves within a very short time period. In this sense, the passage of time would be more relevant. Also, it is probably more likely that significant medical advances will occur over the longer rather than shorter haul, rendering the advance directive less informed than it would be if written closer to the time of when it would be enacted, especially if news of upcoming advances was made public.

such as a power of attorney, that addresses wishes related to future dementia has additional limitations. Persons need to be able to imagine both physical and cognitive changes, including memory impairment. Some people worry that they will "no longer be the same person" and may not experience themselves to be "them." Their transformation might be so drastic as to render previous considerations of the future life to be nothing more than chance guesses.

Let us remember that once someone is deemed incapable, there can in practice be no effective changing of one's mind, other than if the SDM determines that the wishes expressed while capable do not apply in the current situation – and in Ontario, even then, an application must be made to a tribunal, the Consent and Capacity Board, to depart from the wishes (called a "Form E" application). Time does not always permit this to happen. Through writing his wishes (or even had he expressed them verbally) Mr. Black is binding himself in the future to what he presently decides about his future self. Paradoxically, what constitutes an act of freedom to make a choice now for oneself could later also be experienced as imprisonment. In practical terms, the original Mr. Black cannot change his wish after he is deemed incapable to consent to a given treatment, should he wish to reverse his earlier wish. Perhaps post-dementia he does not really care that he can no longer energetically debate with his children. Maybe he has had enough of hiking and prefers to spend most days resting in bed. And perhaps he would want to receive medical treatment even if still he cared about debates and bird watching. Unfortunately, once found to be incapable with respect to a particular decision, Mr. Black cannot confirm his earlier choices, nor can he refute them.[17]

Here we have the crucial distinction between wishes and the many other kinds of decisions we make that also cannot be "undone" or reversed. While we cannot travel backward in time and change the past, outside of our imagination, we can still decide to do something in reaction to a past decision we currently wish we had not made, if we are still deemed capable. We can alter the future to some extent, provided our autonomy is intact. For example, while we cannot reverse the decision to bear a child after the child is born, we can place the child for adoption or surrender the child to a children's welfare agency. There are usually options we can take to continue to exert some control in our life. But with an advance directive expressing a wish to not pursue life-sustaining treatment, there is no further action of self-determination after this one.

(c) Is there only one way to interpret an advance directive?

This question ties in with the irreversibility problem. When we make a decision now about the future, and remain capable, not only can we change our minds but we can also discuss with others what our decisions mean when there

---

[17] In fact, DeGrazia asks if one can neither confirm nor refute an earlier choice, to what extent is it actually an "earlier" choice rather than a "current" one? One could thus argue that there is no precedent autonomy on that basis. One needs a current decision to differentiate it from a former decision or vice versa. See David DeGrazia, "Advance Directives, Dementia, and 'The Someone Else Problem'," *Bioethics* 13, no. 5 (1999): 373–391.

are interpretive problems that involve someone else following our instructions. For example, let us imagine that I am currently a cancer patient. I am reluctant to accept radiation treatment for a variety of reasons, including unwanted side effects. My doctor briefly tells me about treatment X, which has a track record of very few negative effects. I agree to undergo radiation therapy in 2 weeks, as long as radiation treatment X is administered. I consent to no other type. When the treatment time arrives, however, treatment X is not available. The oncologist calls me and asks me what I want to do. He wants me to clarify what I meant when I said I refused all other types of radiation. Did I mean I would accept absolutely no other radiation treatment, but would consent to chemotherapy? Would I be willing to die because I will not accept anything else? He can probe my thinking and ask for clarification about what motivates the decisions I make. I can ask him more questions to be better informed. And, of course, I can change my decision. I might speak to other people who will influence that decision, or I might not. But I am presented with additional opportunities to receive more information and to reflect on what I wish to do.

Mr. Black's advance directive could have raised significant disagreement and moral distress over interpretation. He stated he did not wish to receive treatment if he developed an incurable disease, and he listed the conditions he was referring to. Did he mean that he would not want to be treated for any ailments that could occur parallel to his incurable disease, or did he mean that he refused treatment only for his incurable disease? This key ambiguity is essential to determining whether Mr. Black would have wanted treatment for his pneumonia. Unlike the capable patient who can continue to express her wishes, Mr. Black could not.

(d) Can any of the limitations be overcome or at least improved upon?

In order to counter the difficulty of imagining ourselves to be radically changed by dementia, perhaps we could be exposed to others who either have dementia themselves or have come to learn more about dementia through one means or another. Some ethicists have thought so.[18] For example, we could visit and try to communicate with Alzheimer's patients, their families and the staff members who work with them, read books about the topic, attend lectures, and so forth. Activities such as these might result in increased understanding and might even help us to better imagine ourselves as having a dementia. The concern remains, however, whether we could be sufficiently able to imagine being in this situation to satisfy the requirement of being informed *enough*. Again, we have no clear standard for evaluation. We might feel that the experience of witnessing a loved one's struggle with dementia informs us enough, as perhaps did Mrs. Black. Or we might focus on a different criterion, such as doing academic research on the disease. Given the vagueness of the notion, we really have no objective benchmark to which to refer.

---

[18] See Rebecca Dresser, "Advance Directives in Dementia Research: Promoting Autonomy and Protecting Subjects," IRB: *Ethics and Human Research* 23. no. 1 (2001): 1–6.

On the one hand, there is no such thing as two individuals experiencing dementia in the same way or anticipating their personal experience of it in the future in the same way. On the other hand, I am suggesting we be required to meet a standard of being sufficiently informed. The Ontario laws of consent are fashioned in such a way that there remain only two options: one is either informed or one is not; one is either capable or one is not. In reality, these states are nuanced, not absolute. Often judgment calls are made with regard to the more gray areas. Just exactly when informed turns into "informed enough," especially given the ambiguity around the meanings of "understand" and "appreciate," is anybody's guess as things now stand.

Furthermore, it is difficult for theorists and ethicists to agree upon how much detail and what kind of detail an advance directive should have. If it is too scant, then it is considered too impoverished to understand. If it is very detailed, it might be seen as too cumbersome. I have already referred to Mr. Black's advance directive and the potential interpretation problems that could arise. Perhaps he should have clarified more specifically which diseases warranted treatment and which did not. One could consult a medical encyclopedia disease by disease and still, of course, not be able to consider a future disease that has not yet been identified, much less a cure that might still be discovered. If someone were to write a very extensive description, any scenarios that were not included could mistakenly stand out as overly significant. And as one scholar says, paradoxically, the more information the directive has, the more restrictive it might be in terms of actual applicable situations in real life.[19]

Often, terms are used that are almost absurdly vague, such as "no heroics," "no futile treatment," "life without quality," "suffering too much," etc. These kinds of terms are commonly used in advance directives without reference to underlying values or intentions and thus are open to almost limitless interpretive freedom. Even if an advance directive is clearer, there is still controversy about whether it can ever really encapsulate what the author would want to happen at the time of actual application, due to the predictive problems already discussed. In addition, it is not unusual for patients to change their minds about what kinds of treatments they want.[20] To further complicate matters, some studies conclude that patients do not always want their directives to determine their future treatment.[21] Some would like them to be interpreted and applied with some flexibility.[22] So even if there were some way around the irreversibility of decision and predictive difficulties of advance directives, and we could make

---

[19] Henry S. Perkins, "Controlling Death: The False Promise of Advance Directives," *Annals of Internal Medicine* 147, no. 1 (2007) 51–57.

[20] Dawson, 154.

[21] More on this topic and how substitute decision-makers make use of advance directives will be found in Chap. 4.

[22] Janet Ritchie, Ron Sklar, and Warren Steiner, "Advance Directives in Psychiatry: Resolving Issues of Autonomy and Competence," *International Journal of Law and Psychiatry* 21, no. 3 (1998): 245–260.

them sufficiently informed, we do not even know with confidence that the authors intended to have their wishes taken seriously. And with regard to those who expect *some* latitude will be taken when it comes to interpretation and application of their wishes, how do we translate such a vague expectation into concrete decision-making?

It is vitally important that people remember to review and update advance directives on a regular basis, if at all possible. Sometimes, however, individuals do not even recall having written them. Sometimes, others do not even know about their existence. It is also important to advise SDMs that they have been appointed to this role. It is utterly fascinating to witness the situations where SDMs do not even know they have been named. Of course, it is even better that ongoing discussions occur between the SDMs and the persons in question, so that advance directives can be reviewed together over periods of time, with ample opportunities for discussion, clarification, and possible revisions. It is essential to determine if the SDMs understand what their role is to be and whether it is a duty they are able to fulfill responsibly.

Now, having said that, there is data available indicating that substitute decision-makers do not always abide by the role they are expected to undertake. From my experience, I think that often this is due to a lack of legal understanding about which standard(s) they are to meet, how to determine the meaning of their terms and intent, as well as how to interpret the standards in compliance with the advance directive. I raise this now because there is an argument made that SDMs can always add more "merit" to the advance directive, especially given that we assume the SDMs are apprised of the patients' values and wishes. We must also be careful at this point in time not to assume that compliance with advance directives is necessarily always a good thing for the patients.[23] In fact, I venture to guess that there are times when SDMs do not comply with their legal requirements, because they are uncomfortable with following the standards as they exist and in the order they are meant to be followed.[24] I will return to this point.

With these considerations before us, we can return to a key question posed earlier. I asked whether the identification of the limitations of an advance directive contributes to making the writing of the advance directive more informed. After all, it is a requirement of autonomy and informed consent that the risks be known and appreciated.

Let us say that when Mr. Black wrote his advance directive, he either already knew or was told that he ought to consider the limitations of the advance directive. Perhaps he was told to seriously consider them because the risks of having

---

[23] I am not referring here to the fact that some patients do not wish to have their wishes followed anyway.

[24] We also do not know whether the SDMs who deviate from the legal standards are also ones who were not engaged in discussions earlier on with the patient and thus were not really informed about what the patient wished. There are a variety of potential reasons why SDMs deviate from following the authors' wishes and this topic will be further explored in Chap. 4.

an advance directive are significant. Let us imagine that he was told that not all dementia patients find their lives to be unworthy of living. They may in fact feel quite content. Mr. Black requested refusal of treatment in his directive because he believed at the time of writing the document that he would not want to live with dementia in the future. Suppose also that he was cautioned that his current beliefs about how he would feel in that situation might be wrong and that he should consider this in the formation of his advance directive requests. And imagine that Mr. Black did consider this. Does this mean he is now better informed and thus his advance directive should carry more weight than it would were he not to consider this? And not just consider it, but state in the directive what he wants done if that should happen?

This scenario has been answered by various theorists in the affirmative, with the conclusion that these kinds of considerations constitute additional informa- tion that increases the value of the advance directive.[25] The value lies in the enhancement of understanding the relevant information. Obviously, one must possess information before it can be understood, and the more relevant the information received and considered the better. But, I argue, there is informa- tion of a particular quality that is not enhanced in this way. I am again referring to the concept of "appreciation."

You can tell me a hundred times that I might change my mind later. But I have my mind and emotions, my "now," not my "later" or future mind, nor the benefit of the experience that spans the time between now and then. Giving me additional information of this sort may do very little to assist in my appreciation *now* of how I will feel *later*. I cannot in the present really imagine changing my mind later. The future self-referential problem and experiential gap will likely not be resolved by receipt of more of the same kind of information. Hypothetically, there might be those who would be more open to believing that they might be among those who change their minds. To be truly effective, though, I imagine they would need not only to acknowledge this possibility but to state how they would want their respective SDMs to handle "that situation" should it arise. Once again, we would encounter concerns about how to identify future instances that we can have very little knowledge or appreciation of at this time.

But there is another hypothetical group of advance directive authors I worry more about. They belong to the group who are encouraged to consider that they might be wrong now about what they want in the way of treatment in the future, but unlike the first group, they are not interested in any uncertainties. Their response is different in that they become even more certain that they can currently accurately predict for themselves what they want in the future. Let us imagine Mr. Black to have an amended advance directive that reads something like the follow- ing: "I appreciate that some people with dementia are nonetheless happy and in some sense want to receive treatment. Even if that should be the case for me, I am stating that I still want to receive no treatment in the event that...."

---

[25] DeGrazia, *The Someone Else Problem,* 373–391; Pam R. Sailors, "Autonomy, Benevolence, and Alzheimer's Disease," *Cambridge Quarterly of Healthcare Ethics* 10 (2001): 184–193.

In Mr. Black's case we never got to worry about whether such a clause would be helpful or not, because everyone agreed he was pretty unhappy anyway.

But we could not know what his emotional state would be like in advance. It would seem at first blush that to consider the possibility of "being happy" with dementia in advance and to frame a decision in light of that does seem informed. But I doubt this. If you cannot appreciate a future scenario, you cannot stipulate that your lack of appreciation does not affect what you will, or should, want in that scenario. Identification of an additional scenario does not enhance the value of the directive at all. It perhaps merely fools others into thinking, "Mr. Black was *really* sure he would not want to live with dementia later on, even if he became a "happy person with dementia." He really knew himself then, and he knew then what he would want later, didn't he?"

No, I say. His self-knowledge was unlikely to be especially good at the time of formulating the advance directive, but in any case, no additional thoughts about potential future scenarios, no matter how vivid, how varied, and how specific, would likely help. Additional avowals of confidence in one's abilities of prediction are likely unhelpful. This is a situation where certainty only counts when it is framed in the context of how little one actually knows, not in the context of how much one knows with confidence. Adding content to the directive is different from adding quality. Heaping one unknown upon another does not a robust directive make! It could even hinder someone from reflectively considering that something other than what is written in the directive *then* about *now* ought to be contemplated. And that could result in real harm. This is one of those situations where "knowing how much I don't know" has an advantage, but only if it does not lead me to try to rule out the relevance of the unknowns.

Would I argue similarly if someone wrote in the advance directive that upon becoming "a happy person with dementia," the previous wishes stated in this same advance directive about declining treatment should be overruled? Let us put aside the problem of defining what "a happy person with dementia" might mean and focus exclusively on the question of whether the advance directive now has more merit. Again, from an "understanding" standard point of view, I think this is not unreasonable, though wanting in detail. However, can we say that we can "appreciate" being "a happy patient with dementia" from the present context of being capable? The same arguments apply, so I think the answer, again, is "no." There might seem to be an important difference here. Both advance directive authors may have considered that there are at least two opposing possibilities of emotional experience in the future: being "happy" and being "unhappy,"[26] but only the second one changed her mind about what she would

---

[26] The dichotomy I present is, of course, largely false because people are not either happy or not. I am presenting an extreme oversimplification. If we cannot however resolve these sorts of problems when presented in the extreme, how can we go about applying directives to real-life scenarios where potentially people with dementia express a range of emotions and more than one at a time? How can we capture the continuum of emotional shifts in words of a directive? Because application or refusal of treatment is all or nothing, where do we draw the lines in the shifting sands?

want in terms of future treatment acceptance or refusal as a result. Intuitively, her directive would be better informed than that of the first author. In, fact her directive is as uncritically prescriptive as that of the first author.

The first author allows for the possibility that either experience A ("being miserable") or experience B ("being happy") could happen. In either event, she wishes the outcome to be X (no treatment). She does not differentiate between events A or B in terms of outcome X. The second author also allows for the possibility that either experience A or B could happen. The difference is that in the case of A, she directs that X occur. If she is miserable in the future, she wants no treatment. So far their directives are identical. However, in the event of B ("being happy"), she wants Y (treatment), not X (no treatment). Is this difference significant in terms of the second author's directive being "better informed" and if so, how? The first author chooses the same future outcome regardless of her experience of dementia. The second one chooses her future outcome contingent upon whether or not her experience is a happy one. They are both projecting their current assumptions about what is of value to them into their future decision-making. There really is no reason to assume that one author knows herself currently better than the other author does. There is also no reason to speculate that one is better at making predictions about future experiences or wishes than the other. They are both likely equally deficient when it comes to these matters, just like the rest of us. Nor should their reasons for making these choices matter, because as we know, capable people can make pretty well whatever decisions they want, regardless of how (ir)rational their reasoning appears to be. The concern is that both authors cannot currently appreciate what they might actually appreciate in the future.

I do feel the pull of the idea that the second author's directive is "better." Its merit, however, does not rest in its being any better informed. It is subject to the same type of prediction error as in the case of the other one. Perhaps there is something redeemable in the different outcome, then. How could that be? Surely it is reasonable to be comforted by the fact that due to the idiosyncratic nature of the content of the second author's directive, some future harms are likelier to be avoided. The fact that it allows for the potential continuance of life of a patient with dementia may be a very good thing. It just happens to cohere with what I observe, that is, that it makes intuitive sense to try to prolong a life that, by all accounts, appears to be a happy one, whether there is dementia or not. It has the effect of opting out of the more dominant belief that a life with Alzheimer's cannot be a happy one or one worthy of being extended.[27] But let us remember that in this book, we are focusing on advance directives that stipulate the refusal of treatment. The additional clause is significant only because it

---

[27] We can, of course, never know in advance that acceptance of treatment always ends up to be "good" for the patient. I am circumventing, on purpose, a more inclusive detailing of the difficult navigation around moral and practical issues related to how a "good" is to be defined, how to decide whose opinion gets to count as a "good," and what to do when there are competing multiple "goods." It is impossible to sufficiently address these challenging issues in the scope of this paper. Nonetheless, the case studies I review depict some of the relevant features of the questions above.

has the effect of overriding the refusal. Its merit lies in mitigation of potential harms that are inherent in how advance directives are currently constructed. Surely there are better ways to do this. I will return to this issue. For the moment, I will just say that in the absence of such a kind of advance directive, most people concerned about the hypothetical patient's well-being will likely be biased toward making a decision to help extend her currently happy life.

(e) Do the theorists have anything to say that could help out with any of these limitations?

M.J. Wreen believes that the idea of extending people's ability, to apply their medical treatment decisions at a further time when incapable, is an adequate one in theory, but definitely becomes more challenging when applied in real-life case scenarios.[28] He claims there are a few justifiable exceptions when these decisions should not be honored, including when it is believed that written directives do not comply with what the patients really meant to express, or when the patients did say what they meant to express, but did not consider all the relevant implications involved.[29] I will briefly address both these conditions.

With regard to the former exception, it is reasonable to believe that one could mean to express a particular wish and yet somehow not convey it accurately in written form. For example, perhaps the author hurriedly drafted a vague directive without much thought or without enough details. Or, perhaps so much detail was provided that the gist of it was lost. Another author might have used ambiguous phrases without realizing and so forth.[30] This concern about the difficulties in capturing our desires and directions in written directives is well known. It makes sense to be concerned about honoring such directives. But how would this problem ever come to be known? Clearly, it is only the patients themselves who could have ever known this, because nobody can ever know better than them what it is they want to convey. Some people also are just more certain of what they want to express at any particular point in time and/or are capable of doing a reasonable job of transferring any such wishes into a written form. As well, there may not be others present to guide the process of writing advance directives. If, however, there were others there who were particularly savvy about alerting the authors to take heed of the common problems already mentioned, we cannot escape the fact that in the province of Ontario, directives are not the ultimate stand-alone documents. When it comes time to apply the directives, from a legal point of view, the substitute decision-makers will be interpreting them in order to attempt to apply them to the current medical situations the patients are facing. The interpretation of the directives adds an additional step, in which potentially the difficulty of further deviation from the original wishes of the authors may be compounded. This issue may become

---

[28] M.J. Wreen, "Hypothetical Autonomy and Actual Autonomy: Some Problem Cases Involving Advance Directives," *Journal of Medical Ethics* 15, no. 4 (Winter 2004): 319–333.

[29] Wreen, 319–333.

[30] Olick, 66.

further fraught with uncertainty when there is more than one SDM and, as usually is the case, more than one interpretation being considered.

Wreen's second exception applies when patients have said what they meant to say, but did not consider all the relevant implications involved. It should now be clear that I am hard pressed to identify a situation that, in fact, could be otherwise. Even if we lower the bar to a less strict standard where we expect reasonable consideration of the implications, not perfection, there are usually just too many unknowns for informed decision-making to occur.

Further along in his writings, Wreen states that it is not so much a matter of overriding the advance directives, but rather of trying very hard to determine what, given their values, the patients would have written if they had more thoughtfully considered the matter. He considers it to be a "cognitive oversight" when patients' actual advance directives do not represent their actual interests or values.[31] I think Wreen correctly raises a very important point here when he directs the reader's attention to the authors' values and interests. Oftentimes, the content of advance directives is action-laden as opposed to being illustrative of values and/or interests. Identification of actions divorced from the context of values and interests that render meaning to the directives is highly problematic. The SDMs will be required to make inferences about values and interests drawn from comments about actions. Inferences are subjective in nature, lending greater probability to the likelihood of error. Making errors is not necessarily problematic, as long as they can be remedied. However the SDMs will never know, can never know, if errors are made, because they cannot capably and autonomously confirm with anyone that the inferences made are correct. The inferences are made with reference to past decisions, which also likely compound the probability of error. And the decisions the authors conveyed in the directives are prone to error in the first place, as already discussed. So here we have added an additional layer of difficulty upon difficulty. When we consider that inferences we make every day in real time are fraught with errors, I think it becomes clearer that the SDMs are faced with a task that cannot be performed to the level presupposed for its moral and legal authority.

In Mr. Black's case, no direct mention of his values was present in his advance directive. His advance directive spoke of actions to take in specific scenarios, but we can only guess at what values and beliefs drove his decisions. This difficulty arises in most advance directives that are focused on actions, not on values or beliefs. Unless we can know from Mr. Black directly what his values or beliefs were when he wrote the advance directive, we cannot be in a situation to determine if his stated directions cohere now with his former values. Faced with the interpretation of an advance directive, I often hear the phrase, "But what did he mean when he wrote those words?" Let us see if we can find a way to deduce the values underlying his directives. Do they have to be explicitly written?

Mr. Black indicated that bird watching and hiking with his wife, walking his dogs, having dinner out, and debating with his children were all pleasurable activities. Was it the physical activity part of hiking that was so desirable for

---

[31] Wreen, 319–333.

him? Perhaps it was the challenge of physical exertion or the social aspect. Maybe it was the combination of all of these aspects or the routine of it that he enjoyed the most. It is hard to know with any confidence. We could ask those closest to him to see if they could provide additional information, to help determine what values underlie his choice of these activities. Would we necessarily be better off if we took this approach?

When only activities are listed, as in the case of Mr. Black, how are we to make sense of their coherence with the values of Mr. Black with dementia?[32] If, for example, he was at a stage where he could still hike, though very sporadically and slowly, he could still dine with his wife, meaning they could have their meals together, albeit in the hospital cafeteria, but he could not debate with his children, or would not debate with them, possibly because he no longer seems to have that interest, would we say his same values are current? Would this specific scenario cohere with his desire not to receive treatment? While Mrs. Black is the only attorney for personal care, she still looks to her children for advice. Maybe they would not agree with each other. There is definitely some room for ambiguity and interpretation differences here. Even if they do agree and Mrs. Black feels confident that the situation seems to match what her husband wrote in his advance directive, can we be confident enough that we are identifying the values that Mr. Black was privileging? And even if we could, whether or not these values can be applied to the current Mr. Black with dementia is another issue. What if he changed his values? How would we know? Should that matter? I will argue later that, of course, it should matter. So, even if we were to cast aside all doubts raised due to the problems identified above, how are we to deal with the idea that Mr. Black's values might have changed in the interim?

Concluding Remarks

In the case of Mr. Black, nobody asked if his values had changed. There was no discussion at all about his values. However, if his wife had been concerned that her husband's values had changed significantly since the time he had written the directive, and she felt that he was no longer the "same" person as the one who wrote it,

---

[32] This question assumes that people with dementia are still capable of either maintaining previous values or forming new ones. I agree. I think it is also true that most people with dementia are "valuers," and when I think about this idea, I agree with others that autonomy ought to be understood in this way also. For example, Jaworska claims that values are essential to autonomy and that many Alzheimer's patients are capable of autonomy. See Agnieszka Jaworska, "Respecting the Margins of Agency: Alzheimer's Patients and the Capacity to Value," *Philosophy and Public Affairs* 28, vol. 2 (Spring 1999):105–138. More about the relevance of values will be forthcoming in Chap. 3. There are, though, many ethicists and theorists that do not see autonomy in this way. For example, Ronald Dworkin views autonomy in terms of decision-making capacity and the ability to plan one's life. See Ronald Dworkin, *Life's Dominion: an Argument about Abortion, Euthanasia and Individual Freedom*, (New York: Alfred A. Knopf, 1993).

meaning that his personality seemed to have undergone huge qualitative changes, then it might reasonably follow that there could be questions raised in terms of adhering to it. As Wreen discusses, there could also be further discussion required if there was reason to believe that Mr. Black wrote what he did because he did not consider—probably because he did not know what to consider—all the relevant implications.[33] I appreciate that nobody can know all the relevant implications. However, given that a significant percentage of people with dementia do seem to enjoy quality of life and appear happy much of the time, someone should have given him this information. It is a problem to know who that person ought to be since there is no regulation that some professional or another must even be part of the process of helping someone ponder what should be considered in the writing of an advance directive. Had Mr. Black considered this, he might have requested a different action. And had he indicated in his advance directive that he considered this particular implication, for example, and still arrived at a decision to refuse treatment in the future, then, according to Wreen, his advance directive would carry additional weight than had he not even considered this possibility of seemingly experiencing happiness while having a dementia.[34]

There is something significant in what Wreen is saying here, but again, there is a missing consideration that I have repeatedly emphasized. It is indeed important to consider the possibility that one might end up being a "happy patient with dementia."[35] However, merely thinking about different possibilities does not remove the problem of being able to personally appreciate the experience one would have in the future. I think the experiential gap is just too big. I considered calling this gap an "experiential oversight," but "oversight" implies that one did know and just did not consider whatever should have been considered. But it is not an oversight in this sense, because one could not have appreciated the experience in advance.

Wreen draws our attention to another crucial consideration, which is that the consequences faced when we decide whether or not to honor an advance directive can be life or death.[36] Lack of reasonable certainty about what the person really meant to say in the advance directive, or what the person would have said if all the relevant implications would have been thought through, becomes of even more concern when death might be a consequence or, for that matter, when prolonged suffering might be a consequence.

In thinking about these issues, I consistently ask the following question: if an error is going to be made, which is a "better" error to make? Prolonging someone's suffering when she really wants to be dead or hastening someone's death when she really wants to live? Notice that I am phrasing the question in the present, not in the past. I did not say "wanted to be dead" or "wanted to live" because the whole point of an advance directive is to predict the future time when the treatment would be applied or declined. I think it is fair to say that the point of an advance directive is

---

[33] Wreen, 319–333.

[34] Wreen, 319–333.

[35] Wreen, 319–333.

[36] Wreen, 319–333.

to try to eliminate the existence of both of these errors. I realize that both errors are undesirable, but from a moral point of view, is one "worse" than the other? I do not have an answer for this question. Clearly, though, some others likely would. I would venture to guess that healthcare workers whose trumping value in the face of conflicting values is "above all, save a life" would prefer to avoid the second error, that is, hastening someone's death when the patient really wants to live, because of the possible projection of their own values onto the patient's situation. Some SDMs would do so as well. Again, we are dealing with subjective values of others. This also links to my earlier identification of the role of cultural values and how influential they are in medical decision-making.

In the next chapter, when we review the case of Mrs. Black, the "happy dementia patient", these concerns become more visible and the depth of the challenges presented prove to be more obvious. I will try to determine if there is a viable way to become clearer about knowing if the patient with dementia, Mrs. Black, still has the same preferences she had when she wrote her advance directive. Wreen was concerned whether or not the persons' preferences were actually the ones they meant to convey, and if they considered all the relevant information required, in order to project decision-making into the future.[37] I hope to have demonstrated that while Wreen's ideas are good ones,[38] he has not considered what I think to be two of the most significant flaws of advance directives, and those are the problems of appreciating our subjective experiences in the future, as well as never having the information to be able to consider them in the first place. Worse yet, I think these problems are mostly impossible to resolve. However, I do think he is on the right path in promoting the idea that a focus on values and interests potentially lends merit to the use of advance directives. The question, though, remains whether this approach is sufficient to mitigate the many problems that remain, partly due to the fact that our values may change over time.

Originally, I was planning to present the case of Mr. Black as an example of an advance directive at its best. After all, there did not seem to be any significant problems related to interpretation or application issues. There was mainly decision-making agreement among the SDM and the team at every turn. They were all satisfied that they were "on track" because nobody challenged their thinking. There was no triggering event that alerted them to the possibility that they may have veered away from Mr. Black's wishes due to a variety of reasons as articulated in this chapter.

Probably, when Mr. Black wrote his advance directive, he did not consider, or even realize he should consider, that his substitute decision-maker, may not abide by his wishes in the advance directive. We cannot however know if she interpreted his advance directive according to how he meant it to be interpreted. He probably did not know that on many occasions, (for a variety of reasons) SDMs do not follow the wishes of directives. Even if he did have this general information to consider, he would have been faced with the appreciation issue that we have already addressed.

---

[37] Wreen, 319–333.
[38] Wreen, 319–333.

Even if we were to allow for the possibility that he could have appreciated this information, he would not be able to predict whether or not this kind of compliance problem would apply to his personal situation.

Perhaps when Mr. Black wrote his advance directive, he did not intend for his wife to follow his wishes exactly as stated. Perhaps he was expecting that she would likely deviate somewhat, be it in terms of timing of its application and/or from a content point of view. Perhaps this was even a desirable expectation for him, and, knowing his wife as he did, he predicted to himself that she likely would. And perhaps she lived up to his expectation. Maybe he did not even care if, in the end, she did not comply at all with it. We just cannot know any of this with any confidence.

Sources

Dawson, Angus. "Advance Directives." In *General Practice and Ethics*, edited by Christopher Dowrich and Lucy Fritch, 130–171. London: Rutledge, 1999.

DeGrazia, David. "Advance Directives, Dementia, and 'The Someone Else Problem.'" *Bioethics* 13, no. 5 (1999): 373–391.

Dresser, Rebecca. "Advance Directives in Dementia Research: Promoting Autonomy and Protecting Subjects." *IRB: Ethics and Human Research* 23, no. 1 (Jan–Feb 2001): 1–6.

Dworkin, Ronald. *Life's Dominion: An Argument about Abortion, Euthanasia, and Individual Freedom*. New York: Alfred A. Knopf, 1993.

Freedman, Benjamin. "Informed Consent and the Competent Patient." In *Readings in Biomedical Ethics: a Canadian Focus*. 2nd ed. Edited by Eike-Henner W. Kluge, 169–181. Scarborough: Prentice Hall, 1999.

Holstein, M.B. "Ethics and Alzheimer's Disease: Widening the Lens." *Journal of Clinical Ethics* 9, no. 1 (1998): 13–22.

Jaworska, Agnieszka. "Respecting the Margins of Agency: Alzheimer's Patients and the Capacity to Value." *Philosophy and Public Affairs* 28, vol. 2 (Spring 1999): 105–138.

Olick, Robert S. "On the Scope and Limits of Advance Directives and Prospective Autonomy." In *Advance Directives*, edited by P. Lack, N. Biller-Andorno and S. Brauer. New York: Springer Press, 2014.

Perkins, Henry. "Controlling Death: The False Promise of Advance Directives." *Annals of Internal Medicine* 147, no. 1 (2007): 51–57.

Ritchie, Janet, Sklar, Ron and Steiner, Warren. "Advance Directives in Psychiatry: Resolving Issues of Autonomy and Competence." Journal of Law and Psychiatry 21, no. 3 (1998): 245–260.

Sailors, Pam R. "Autonomy, Benevolence, and Alzheimer's Disease." *Cambridge Quarterly of Healthcare Ethics* 10 (2001): 184–193.

Thiel, Mary-Jo. "Personal Capacity to Anticipate Future Illness and Treatment Preferences". In *Advance Directives,* edited by P. Lack, N. Biller-Andorno and S. Brauer, 21. New York: Springer Press, 2014.

Wreen, M.J. "Hypothetical autonomy and actual autonomy: some problem cases involving advance directives." *Journal of Medical Ethics* 15, no. 4 (Winter 2004): 319–333.

Chapter 3
Mrs. Black

In this chapter, I will discuss the case of Mrs. Black. In many important ways, her situation is very similar to that of her late husband, Mr. Black. There is, however, at least one crucial difference: Mrs. Black seems to be very content with her current life, even though she has dementia.[1] A particularly interesting prospect is that, in part, her contentedness is *caused* by her dementia.

Mrs. Black

Mrs. Black is an 85-year-old woman with mid-stage Alzheimer's disease. During the past 3 years, she has been living in a long-term care facility on a unit that provides care to dementia residents. Here is how Mrs. Black's medical staff and care providers would characterize the state of her illness and her emotional life, based on their familiarity with her: While able to walk on her own, she requires assistance with grooming, hygiene, and feeding, which she graciously accepts. When seated at the window in her room, she is content to cast her gaze outside, and occasional shrieks of delight are heard when birds pass by. She loves music and continuously plays the same Frank Sinatra songs, often singing along. Mrs. Black attends most of the recreational and social programs and is often observed to be smiling, clapping, and hugging other residents, irrespective of whether she knows them. Her level of cognition is variable. When asked questions such as "Would you like your tea now?", sometimes her only response is to stare back and smile. She derives great

---

[1] See Andrew Firlik's discussion about the case of Margo, where he considers the idea that dementia might interfere with the worries arriving at the brain. Andrew Firlik, "A Piece of My Mind: Margo's Logic," *Journal of the American Medical Association*, no. 265 (1991): 191. Also see Maarthe Schermer, "In search of 'the good life' for demented elderly," *Medicine, Health Care and Philosophy*, no. 6 (2003): 35. Schermer notes that some persons with dementia appear happy and tranquil, and I confirm this belief as well, based upon my own observations.

© Springer International Publishing AG 2018
M. Sokolowski, *Dementia and the Advance Directive*,
https://doi.org/10.1007/978-3-319-72083-8_3

pleasure from leafing through the same two or three magazines, propped upside down in her lap.[2]

For the past several months, the only person she consistently recognizes is her attendant nurse, whom she fondly greets by name. When close relatives visit, initially Mrs. Black does not recognize them. Nonetheless, she greets them warmly and politely asks who they are. Flashes of recognition appear on her face when they respond. After several minutes, she often appears confused and again asks them to introduce themselves. This is a pattern that reoccurs. Nonetheless, it is apparent that Mrs. Black rejoices in their company. She is rarely embarrassed or frustrated by her lapses of memory. Perhaps she no longer remembers that she forgets. Mrs. Black is one of the happiest residents with dementia that I have ever met.

Mrs. Black's husband died 5 years ago in a rehabilitation unit of a hospital. He had written an advance directive, and, shortly after his death, she decided to write one too. Her son reported that she had done so based upon her belief that her husband's directive had proven very useful to her family and the medical team, at a time when Mr. Black was unable to express his wishes and the physician was recommending the insertion of a feeding tube.

Mrs. Black's advance directive stipulated that if she were to suffer any medical condition that resulted in her not being able to recognize her family members, and if the medical condition was not reversible, she would not wish to receive any medical treatment, except for pain control, and would want to be allowed to die, if that should be the consequence.

Mrs. Black enjoyed general good health, aside from her dementia, until a week ago when she suddenly developed a high fever accompanied by vomiting and drowsiness. Her physician, Dr. Swift, told her she may have contracted a very serious bacterial infection. He informed her that without intravenous antibiotics, she would likely soon die. Mrs. Black smiled at him and pointed to the wall. Dr. Swift attempted twice more to explain the dire situation to obtain consent to medical treatment at this point in time, to no avail. Aware that her son Robert, an optometrist living in a rural area about two hours away, was her substitute decision-maker, Dr. Swift contacted him to inform him about his mother's current medical situation and the proposed treatment plan. After explaining the risks and benefits of the antibiotic regime, he sought Robert's consent. Robert refused. Puzzled by this response, Dr. Swift reiterated that, without aggressive antibiotic treatment, Robert's mother would likely soon die. Robert again refused. Dr. Swift was bewildered. He called an emergency team meeting and urged Robert to attend.

---

[2] While I am accepting the team's psychological ascriptions of Mrs. Black's medical team more or less at face value, given the plausibility that they have reliable insights about their most familiar clients and patients, I also recognize that there is much controversy about the ascription of complex thoughts and emotions to persons who are inexpressive or expressively "incoherent." This issue is complex and is best left to philosophy of mind and philosophy of language scholars for in-depth discussions, an ambitious undertaking that is beyond the scope of this book.

Robert informed the team that his mother had completed an advance directive a few years ago. They had been unaware of its existence.[3] He explained that his father had also an advance directive and that his mother felt it had served them all well, providing clarity about his wishes when he was unable to express himself. Robert distributed copies for the team to review. He insisted that his mother's situation reflected the conditions she specified in her directive. He reviewed her medical status as was explained to him by the medical staff. His mother was diagnosed with Alzheimer's disease, an irreversible disease, and she was currently not able to recognize her family members. She now required treatment for her illness. According to her directive, treatment other than pain control was to be refused.

Yet some team members wondered if Mrs. Black had meant her words to be taken so literally. Robert affirmed it to have been his mother's intent in authorizing the advance directive. He also reminded the team that his mother had chosen him as her legal attorney for personal care, and therefore, it was his obligation to fulfill that role responsibly. He implored the team to immediately establish a care plan that would provide his mother with a "most comfortable death." A long silence followed.

The entire medical team was devastated. The staff members fervently believed that if Mrs. Black was currently able to express herself, she would consent to receive treatment to try to prolong her life. In fact, they insisted that her seemingly happy demeanor was an expression of just that. In their view, her advance directive did not reflect her current wishes. Given her zeal for life, her daily enjoyment of recreational activities, and her love of social contact, they felt it would have been "completely unethical" to withhold treatment. They felt it was wrong to comply with the wishes of her advance directive. To do so, most expressed, would be tantamount to "murdering" her. An intensely emotional discussion followed. Team members, including the medical unit's social worker, explicitly lamented that she had ever written an advance directive, which in some team members' opinions amounted to little more than "legalese jargon." The unit manager contended that without an advance directive, Mrs. Black would probably have been receiving treatment today.[4]

Lilly, the nurse expressed doubt about the legitimacy of the directive. Mrs. Black, she hypothesized, created it shortly after her husband's death at a time when, in all likelihood, she was both depressed and unduly influenced by her husband's potential desolate experience of living with dementia. Mr. Black's alleged depressed state, she emphasized, was a very different reality than was the joyful mood Mrs. Black was experiencing. Lilly surmised when Mrs. Black wrote the directive she probably did not consider (or know to consider) the idea that she could have a

---

[3] The usual practice at this particular facility is for the team clerk to inquire about the existence of an advance directive at the time the intake forms are completed. After admission, the advance directive is kept in the patient's file. In this particular case, upon review it was discovered that the usual team clerk was absent on the day in question, and the substitute staff member mistakenly overlooked this particular duty.

[4] In the absence of any known previous capable wishes, Ontario laws would require a best interest standard to be followed. Doing so may very well have resulted in giving Mrs. Black the treatment. *Health Care Consent Act*, S.O. 1996 c. 2, Sched. A, s. 59 (1).

dementia and still enjoy a good quality of life.[5] Therefore, Lilly concluded, it would be wrong to solely rely on the contents of a document that Mrs. Black had never updated and presently could neither refute nor confirm. "Mrs. Black is one of the happiest persons I know," she insisted, "and that is *the* relevant factor the decision should rest upon."[6] Additionally, one of the nurse assistants, Mary, argued that Mrs. Black had changed so much during the past few years that she was "no longer the same person" with the same values. "It is a violation of who she is now to refer back to her wishes of so many years ago." Other staff members nodded in agreement.

Nonetheless, Robert insisted that it was his duty to act on the basis of his mother's previous wishes. After all, she had expressed great relief after she completed her directive, comforted by the belief that her wishes would be followed. He reminded the team that he (and his sisters) know his mother the best and that her current state of happiness did not count as a reason to ignore her directive.[7] He threatened a lawsuit if the team did not immediately act in compliance with its terms.

---

[5] Dresser advocates that persons writing an advance directive be as informed as possible about Alzheimer's disease including its various stages. It is very possible that Mrs. Black did not receive sufficient information, including the knowledge that some patients with Alzheimer's disease live happy lives. Rebecca Dresser, "Advance Directives in Dementia Research: Promoting Autonomy and Protecting Subjects," *IRB: Ethics and Human Research* 23, no. 1 (Jan–Feb 2001): 2.

[6] Lilly claimed that the perceived happiness of the patient was *the* relevant factor for decision-making. However, she also claimed that we ought not to have *solely* depended on the contents of her advance directive, in part because of the irreversibility problem inherent to all directives of this nature, in part due to potential lack of information (she probably did not know to consider she might in the future have what appears to be an overall happy life as opposed to an unhappy one), and in part due to the influences of her likely depressed mood at the time she wrote her advance directive. So it appears to me that she was prepared to give some consideration to the advance directive. If Mrs. Black had considered the idea that she might be "a happy patient with dementia," and still wanted her advance directive to have full force, would that have resulted in Lilly holding onto the claim that she ought to receive treatment? Did Lilly mean that the state of happiness was the *most* relevant factor? She could not have literally meant it to be the *only* relevant factor or she would not have even considered the advance directive. Given that some features of the advance directive that Lilly criticized are indigenous to all directives (irreversibility, lack of information and appreciation), nonetheless, she must have thought that there was something potentially useful about them to warrant some consideration. Whatever they may have been, they were less "weighty" in terms of importance than was the perceived state of happiness, in terms of decision-making. It seemed to me that Lilly started off with the default position of use of the advance directive, but then discounted its overall value in comparison to Mrs. Black's current state of happiness. However, she did indicate that the ultimate decision ought to be based upon something *in addition* to the advance directive. It is possible that she felt that the advance directive potentially could have been one of the relevant factors in decision-making if it could have met a certain threshold of "value" and had that been the case that it would have been either competing with or cohering with currently perceived wishes of the patient. If the former happens to be the case, which it likely was in this situation, then "happiness" wins out. We do not know though that "state of (un)happiness" would have been the trumping factor if the situation was reversed. For example, if the advance directive had stated that she would like to receive all possible life-saving treatments, and if Mrs. Black so happened to become an unhappy person with dementia would Lilly have argued that we ought not to try to save her life?

[7] His sisters were living abroad and were not designated as attorneys for personal care.

Dr. Swift asked Robert to allow the team to meet alone for a period of time. As soon as Robert left, expressions of panic and moral distress filled the room. One nurse started to cry, while others angrily protested against Robert's demand. Dr. Swift stated that they had no other choice but to reluctantly agree to do what the son had ordered. After all, Mrs. Black had written an advance directive and her son was fulfilling his legal duty to ensure it would be followed. Dr. Swift noted that while there was a legal option they could pursue that might result in being allowed to provide Mrs. Black with antibiotics, the likelihood of a positive outcome was very small. He empathized with their sadness and agreed that "treating her would definitely be the moral thing to do," expressing his frustration with the gap between morality and the law. He announced he was going to order comfort measures for Mrs. Black and tried to prepare them for the inescapability of her imminent death. The attending nurse said she would feel like a murderer if Mrs. Black continued in her care, and she arranged for a colleague to take her place. She stated, emotionally, that the withholding of treatment in this particular case was contrary to the core nursing values she stood for.

Mrs. Black died 3 days later, most likely due to a fatal bacterial infection. While her son was at peace with the outcome, the team members continued to experience a high level of moral distress over the ensuing few weeks. In general, they felt that, legalities aside, they did not act in accordance with their professional duties, as they understood them to be.[8] In particular, most felt they had violated their overriding professional principle, "Do No Harm." They bemoaned the fact that Mrs. Black was robbed of the chance to live happily for an additional number of years. While the entire team was distraught by the circumstances of her death, a few specifically felt like they were accessories to a crime. "My hands are tainted with her blood" is how one staff member described her shame and guilt. Many of the staff members had developed very close relationships with Mrs. Black over the past 4 years, and her death under these circumstances compounded their grief.

Discussion and Analyses

One issue shared between Mr. and Mrs. Black's cases is whether the advance directive met the criteria for informed consent. The question of what we ought to do when the current wishes, values, or interests of Mrs. Black conflict with those expressed in her advance directive is one of the most compelling issues of all. The topic of values was introduced in the last chapter as well. In this chapter, I will argue for the preeminent role of values and valuation in decision-making with respect to determining treatment for people in Mrs. Black's position. In the end, I recommend

[8] In all likelihood they all appreciated that acting professionally entailed acting according to the purview of the law. I do not mean to imply otherwise. They seemed to be acutely aware that there was a perceived great divide between their legal responsibilities and professional practice duties.

a few specific ways of rethinking the moral status and use of the advance directive, including, of course, the one created by Mrs. Black.

As we did with Mr. Black's case, let's consider some of the key ethical and conceptual issues related to the case of Mrs. Black.[9]

Did Mrs. Black's Advance Directive Meet the Criteria of Informed Consent?

(a) As we know, an important part of the informed consent process in the context of proposed treatment is disclosure of relevant information.

We have no information about whether or not Mrs. Black had any medical input in her decision-making. Directives that are undertaken with the support of a physician might result in increased merit of the directive.[10] However, as mentioned in Chap. 2, having someone available who could appropriately assist the author of the directive by offering a clinical perspective is neither a legal requirement nor necessarily a common reality. In Ontario, the *Substitute Decisions Act*, 1992, S.O. 1992, c. 30, sets a threshold for capacity to sign a power of attorney for personal care (a form of wishes). Section 47 creates the legal test as follows, and it is focused on ability to understand and to appreciate who will become the proposed attorney and the role they will assume; not the nature or quality of the decisions they will be required to make:

47 (1) A person is capable of giving a power of attorney for personal care if the person,

(a) has the ability to understand whether the proposed attorney has a genuine concern for the person's welfare; and
(b) appreciates that the person may need to have the proposed attorney make decisions for the person.

We also do not know if it was (sufficiently) explained to Mrs. Black that if she subsequently changed her mind about any of the treatment wishes expressed in her directive, she would be required to be deemed capable at this later date when she might wish to change her original instructions. Nor do we know whether she considered, or even knew to consider, that most persons are not good predictors of what they might want for themselves in the future. Her directive may well have amounted to nothing more than a standard legal form that she just signed, unaided, and basically uninformed. Of course, it is possible that Mrs. Black had engaged in a thoughtful process

---

[9] A more comprehensive review and analysis of the role of the SDM will be undertaken in Chap. 4.

[10] I say "might" because it will very much depend on the individual physician's knowledge of the disease, as well as how much information is shared by the physician, what information the physician thinks is relevant to share, and the extent to which there is disclosure of risks, benefits, and consequences of treatment types, etc.

when she authored the contents and was at least somewhat informed. But the paucity of such good information and of standard procedures for generating appropriately careful reflection makes this prospect inherently unlikely.[11]

It is reasonable to doubt that Mrs. Black was aware that some people with dementia live very happy lives. But in any case, we do not know whether she possessed this information.[12] While her son told the team she went through a "thorough process" when she wrote her advance directive, we do not know specifically what he meant nor was he willing to share more information with us about that. In any event, having the information shared with you is one thing. Being sufficiently informed also requires being able to understand all the relevant information.[13]

(b) The question related to Mrs. Black's appreciation of whatever information she did possess is a crucial one. In her advance directive, Mrs. Black refers to a potential future situation where she might contract an irreversible disease that would result in her inability to recognize other people. Alzheimer's dementia is one pathology that fits this description. In the previous chapter, I discussed the challenge of predictive moral imagination. As I argued in that chapter, I do not believe that is possible. In Mrs. Black's case, this latter concern became a huge problem later on given the imminent risks she faced by refusing treatment (as expressed in her advance directive). If she had been able to truly appreciate the consequences, would that have changed what she thought she might want in terms of accepting or declining treatment or impacted her decision about whether or not she ought to write an advance directive? Again, we do not know.

(c) Was Mrs. Black depressed when she wrote her advance directive?

Nobody questioned her emotional state at the time. I think the question is an important one, likely to generalize to many other cases. In fact, a team member

---

[11] I am oversimplifying here by presenting these two extremes to make a point. At the end of the day, however, I am doubtful that the distinction between these two scenarios is of value. In other words, there is only so much one can do to try to bolster the utility value of a directive, such as giving the contents thorough consideration, and being significantly informed about the limitations, etc. As discussed previously in Chap. 2, the concept of an advance directive and the current (legally driven) application standards are so flawed that I am of the opinion that those efforts are, at best, likely very limited, if, not altogether futile.

[12] Neither do we know if this piece of information has significant relevance for Mrs. Black. Here we are again entering into the topic of what specific information would be considered "reasonable" to impart to someone in her situation. In my opinion, this is an example of a piece of information that she ought to have received. Whether it is applicable to her personal values and beliefs is something for her to decide.

[13] Informed consent studies, historically, have paid little attention to information processing and the possibility that over-disclosure is as frequent an occurrence as is under-disclosure of relevant information. I have heard patients complain that their practitioners inundated them with a great deal of medical information that they did not understand within a short period of time, and at a time when a medical diagnosis or treatment was being explained, generally a time fraught with much anxiety for them. I agree that this particular dynamic is problematic and deserving of more attention, particularly in terms of how it can best be remediated. See Tom L. Beauchamp and James F. Childress, *Principles of Biomedical Ethics*, 2nd ed. (New York: Oxford University Press, 1983), 83.

did subsequently worry that Mrs. Black was likely mourning the death of her husband at the time she wrote her directive. If she was depressed, then it would have been advisable to further assess whether her emotional state was interfering with her ability to understand the information being presented to her about advance directives and to appreciate the consequences. This becomes a moot point today in the sense that we do not have any recourse to take in order to establish what her mental status was at that particular time.

(d) Was Mrs. Black already suffering from a mild form of Alzheimer's when she completed her advance directive?

Nobody raised this question. Yet it is not too far-fetched a consideration given that Mrs. Black wrote her advance directive 5 years ago and she was diagnosed with Alzheimer's disease just 1 year later. She may have had the beginnings of the disease somewhat in advance of its being diagnosed. It may have been prudent to try to access her medical records (with consent, if legally she could meet its criteria) to establish how advanced her dementia was at the time of diagnosis. However, even if she was heading toward the moderate stage, we cannot surmise that she had significant impairment when she wrote her directive. Even if that happened to be the case, we cannot conclude that she was unable to meet the criteria of informed consent. Indeed, in my experience, it is not rare for medical workers to think that most people are first motivated to consider writing an advance directive when they experience some impairment of memory or other cognitive ability. Let's imagine for a moment that we were able to access Mrs. Black's medical records (again, with consent) and learned she had likely suffered from mild stage Alzheimer's for a couple of years by then. That information would raise the possibility that she was at least mildly cognitively impaired when she wrote her advance directive. It is possible that she may not have been able to meet the legal standard of capacity to do so at that time.[14] Paradoxically, however, the experience of dementia that may have rendered her legally incapable could also have made it easier for her to relate to the decisions she was advancing and thus be better able to understand and/or appreciate the consequences. This topic will be more fully explored in the next chapter in the case of Mr. White.

(e) Is Mrs. Black's advance directive potentially better informed because of her past experience with the one her husband wrote?

It could be argued that Mrs. Black had the benefit of experience in the sense that her late husband had previously written an advance directive and she felt that it had served her husband well. There may have been other benefits she perceived to be forthcoming based upon her experience with her husband's directive. The interests of the family and team members may have been served

---

[14] However, there is tremendous individual variation in how the disease affects persons, both from a symptom point of view and the speed of regression. It is also very possible that in a significant number of cases, persons with early dementia could meet the legal standard of informed consent. As well, the content of some advance directives would require less sophisticated reasoning abilities than would others.

by them believing that they were in compliance with his advance directive and thus had honored his wishes.[15] The existence of an advance directive is often perceived to be of benefit to family members and practitioners who may feel relieved of the usual anguish they would otherwise have felt when facing very difficult end-of-life decisions in the absence of an advance directive.

Let us assume that, broadly speaking, similar kinds of prediction problems and the difficulties of not having sufficient relevant information and experience required to make an informed decision were operating more or less equally across both cases. Mr. Black may not have been any better a predictor of what he would want in a future state with dementia than was Mrs. Black.[16] However, as it just so happens, Mr. Black was an unhappy person with dementia, while Mrs. Black was not. In her situation, there were two conflicts of interest, one between what she anticipated her dementia experience would be and the reality of it, which is pretty clearly a mismatch, and one between the wishes she expressed in the advance directive on the basis of that prediction and her current wishes, which is conceptually a more difficult claim because it rests on the idea that Mrs. Black has wishes in her dementia state comparable to those she had in her pre-dementia state. Whatever she loses subsequently in terms of the cognitive connections and rational faculties that would normally situate one's thoughts about the livability of one's life, she at least gains a more direct knowledge of the life she is evaluating. If Mrs. Black, at the time when she wrote her advance directive, had more psychologically normal wishes, she also plausibly suffered from a serious ignorance about the life she was judging to be not worth living. In the case of Mr. Black, what he wrote in his advance directive seemed more aligned with his best interests as a patient with dementia than was the case with Mrs. Black. It is not unlikely that had Mr. Black not had an advance directive, his best interests might well have been perceived by the medical team to be very similar to what he did write in his directive.

---

[15] I admit that my comments regarding the serving of interests are oversimplified. They read as if interests are either served or not, while in reality they are obviously much more nuanced and complex. In Chap. 4 I will present a more robust description and analysis.

[16] It is equally plausible that Mr. Black was a better predictor than was Mrs. Black. However, on an individual case-by-case situation, we cannot with confidence say that one specific person is more competent at prediction than another. Nor can we predict who will be better predictors, as far as I know anyway. Limitations regarding future treatment options probably apply more or less the same across the general nonmedical public. However, one may know oneself better than the other does, and in this sense one may have an advantage over the other. There are additional elements of influence to be considered, such as how much information the author received from reliable sources about potential future treatments.

In What Way Is Mrs. Black's "Happiness" Relevant?

There was a high degree of confidence among the staff members, primarily due to Mrs. Black's elevated spirits and zest for life, that if she could currently express herself verbally, she would opt to have treatment that would hopefully extend her life. In fact, they argued that most of her actions and expressions were "telling us in her way" that she wanted to go on living. Sadly, unless she was going to receive the requisite treatment, her death would be imminent.

Her son argued that it is irrelevant that his mother was happy.[17] He explained that her prior wishes were made without consideration of her future emotional mood(s) not because she failed to give it thought, but rather because it did not factor as important to her then. Was "happiness" something that Mrs. Black considered through most of her life to be of little importance to her? Regardless, it could be true that in her current life, her experience of joy was something of significant value to her. We do not know if the considerations her son raises that reflect her past are relevant ones for her currently. The important topic of coherence of values in advance directives with those existing today will be addressed in an upcoming section.

What Should We Do Given That The Post-Dementia Wishes, Values or Interests of Mrs. Black Seemed to Conflict with Those of Her Advance Directive?

(a) Framing the debate

Most of the literature on advance directives over the past 25 years or so centers on something like this question: Should current "incapable" wishes of the (nonautonomous) dementia patient override previous capably expressed wishes of the pre-dementia (autonomous) person?[18] Usually, the debate is framed in

---

[17] In this case, currently the patient happens to be a very happy one and it is not unusual for others to make the inferential leap that goes something like this: "she has a good quality of life, and most people with a good quality of life want to continue to live, so therefore, it is prudent to give her treatment with the hope of prolonging her life." What if she was happy roughly half the time? What if she was happy only on Fridays? What amount of happiness (never mind the question of how to define the concept) would qualify as meeting the criteria for a good enough life that ought to be continued? Who gets to make that judgment? You can see that again we are dealing with very subjective values and beliefs that get played out in the interpretations that others are making on the patient's behalf and that influence the kinds of decisions they argue for with regard to medical treatment. Interestingly, Newton argues that the notion of contentment is irrelevant. See Michael J. Newton, "Precedent Autonomy: Life-Sustaining Intervention and the Demented Patient," *Cambridge Quarterly of Healthcare Ethics* 8, no. 2 (April 1999): 190.

[18] Jakov Gather and Jochen Bollmann, "How to Decide? Evaluating the Will of a Person with Dementia in the Light of Current Behavior, Advance Directive and Legal Representatives' Perspectives", GeoPsych 28, no. 1 (2015): 19. These authors describe a case where they argue

"all or nothing" absolute terms. The patient is understood to be "capable" or "incapable" and "autonomous" or "nonautonomous" and is referred to as the "then" person versus the "now" person. The debate is set up in such a way as to imply that there are two mutually exclusive and predetermined options, only one of which can be right.[19] The tendency to frame the discussions in such extreme terms stems from the legal frameworks and subsequent healthcare policies that practitioners are obliged to follow. The debate is worded in such a way that it oversimplifies the issues and does not capture the nuances and complexities that exist. For example, in reality, competencies are often partial. They usually fluctuate and represent a range of ability areas. While Alzheimer's is a degenerative and terminal disease roughly characterized by three stages, mild, moderate, and severe, its course does not present as a steady, even decline. As I will address in more detail later on, some competencies may remain quite intact throughout, while others wax and wane. And of course, there is no sharp transition between a "then" person and a "now" person; this distinction is an explicit idealization.

(b) Reframing the debate

I prefer my open-ended version of framing the ethical issue: "What should we do given that the current wishes, values, or interests of Mrs. Black seem to conflict with those of her advance directive?" This does not assume an either/or approach nor depend on polarized terms. For this reason, it does not predetermine the available options to the same extent as the traditional framework. In particular, the reframed question does not assume that the wishes of those with Alzheimer's are incompetent just because they are not characteristic of the clearest non-pathological cases of competent decision-making nor does it exclude the possibility that patients such as Mrs. Black have interests and values

---

against undermining patient's authority by "putting an earlier autonomous expression of the will on a level with a nonautonomous expression of will that is highly open for interpretation."

[19] It is also common to hear the term "previous or former wishes." What is meant when we say this? Do we mean that wishes are prior to the onset of dementia? Or do we mean that wishes are previous to current wishes? As far as I can tell, there are two general ways that we can understand the term "previous or former wishes." The first way it is used refers to the time before either the patient was diagnosed with dementia or before the patient lost the requisite autonomy or capacity to make an informed treatment decision. It unrealistically depicts a rigid boundary between "before" and "after" that does not exist and does not acknowledge any gradations. Changes are usually more subtle and fluctuating in nature. The second and less common way speaks directly to the question about whether or not the current patient with dementia holds the same wishes now that were held in the past when the directive was written. I prefer to use the term according to the second use. I have several reasons. Firstly, it gets away from the thinking that what really matters most is whether the person has dementia or not and relies less upon the existence of a pathological disease being the determining event in whether or not the patient's previous wishes get to count as having value when it comes to adherence to treatment decisions or wishes. It also gets us out of the usual rut of conflating capacity with autonomy and with personhood, meaning that to have capacity is have autonomy and vice versa. It moves us away from the idea that to count as a full person with decision-making capacities is to be autonomous and/or capable and so on. It no longer implies that having a dementia such as Alzheimer's means that your status as a person is diminished.

simply because they are less than stereotypical examples of interests and values.

(c) Law and clinical reality: the great divide

While the law pertaining to medical decision-making does not recognize partial intelligence (or other kinds of intelligence related to emotions, social knowledge, spirituality, and religion), nor even partial autonomy for that matter, these characterizations cohere better with what I have observed to be the case for patients with Alzheimer's disease. It is impossible to apply the legal frameworks to real-life human situations without feeling that a cookie cutter method is being used and that this method just does not work. The reality is that these situations are unique in significant ways, the variations among them substantial. Let me try to explain this more succinctly in the context of the case of Mrs. Black. Since Mrs. Black was unable to understand the information about the treatment that was being offered to her post-dementia, nor able to appreciate the reasonably foreseeable consequences of the risks and benefits for herself,[20] she was deemed incapable (and nonautonomous) from a legal point of view. While the context of using these labels is supposed to be decision-specific (and attributable to that specific time), they are unfortunately perceived by a number of healthcare providers to be applicable to dementia patients in a more generalized way.

One reason for this is that a significant percentage of healthcare providers are uninformed, or positively misinformed, about the legal definition of capacity. I suspect that another reason is attributable to lack of knowledge about how the disease can affect different brain areas, resulting in some areas and hence some capacities being more compromised than others. As well, there is significant variation in how the disease manifests itself from person to person.

Let us also remember that when it comes to healthcare law, autonomy is defined in terms of autonomous actions, as opposed to what qualities define an autonomous person and is furthermore construed rather narrowly as a mere decision-making capacity. One is autonomous according to the law if and only if one can make treatment capacity decisions and the concepts are interdependent and even inter-defined.[21] The legal concept of competence is likewise narrowly defined into a "hypercognitive" view.[22] This sense of capacity appeals

---

[20] See Ontario's *Health Care Consent Act*, 1996, c.2, Schedule A, s. 4 (1).

[21] And bear in mind that it is also a very partial or specific kind of restrained autonomy because it is the practitioners who do the selecting of which kinds of treatment their patients will be offered. The values and beliefs of the respective practitioners, influenced in part by social/professional conditioning, will obviously limit what treatment options are decided to be offered or not.

[22] A term used by Post and O'Neill. This term is meant to convey a disdain for a very narrow understanding of how to determine a person's worth, capacity and ability to direct their own lives. In their opinion and in mine, it does not capture the breadth of these concepts, but relegates worth only to the arena of specific mental aptitudes required for medical decision-making. See Stephen G. Post, "Respectare: Moral Respect for the Lives of the Deeply Forgetful," in *Dementia: Mind, Meaning and the Person*, ed. Julian C. Hughes, Stephen J. Louw and Steven R. Sabat (Oxford: Oxford University Press, 2006), 223; and Desmond O'Neill, "Cogito Ergo Sum? Refocusing

only to the abilities required to make specific medical treatment decisions involving understanding all the relevant information and appreciation of the consequences. Astonishingly, Ontario's *Health Care Consent Act* is silent on what the terms "understanding" and "appreciation" are meant to convey here. No doubt this is a key element explaining the fact that, as already noted, these concepts are often interpreted very subjectively and differently from one practitioner or medical team to the next.

The team has to somehow square this legal conception of the patient as incapable and nonautonomous, and thus not legally recognized as a person who can make medical treatment decisions (specific to the ones she is incapable and nonautonomous to make at a particular time), with the person/patient in front of them who they have come to know in a much fuller way.

Obviously, there are huge implications for calling someone "nonautonomous" or, interchangeably, "incapable" in healthcare organizations. Mrs. Black is a great case in point. Because she did not meet the legal criteria for capacity to decide if she wanted to accept treatment or not, the autonomy standard as entailed in Ontario's *Health Care Consent Act* requires us to then try to determine what her most recent prior capable wishes were, applicable to the current situation. In Mrs. Black's case, they were contained in her advance directive.

(d) What is wrong with this scenario?

For starters, you can see how morally distressing this was for the whole team and understandably so. Moral distress is not to be taken lightly and can have quite devastating effects on the team. Equally, if not more distressing, is that medical decision-making that was done according to narrow legal standards would have implications for whether or not Mrs. Black would receive treatment that would keep her alive and that would allow her to continue to enjoy her current life. The team members were caught between their requirement to follow legal standards and their own professional standards of "doing good" and, above all, "doing no harm." Doing "good" does not just relate to following the patient's wishes but also to doing what is in the best interests of the patient. However, the first legal standard one is required to apply is autonomy (and, as we already know, a very narrow view of it). Since Mrs. Black was *now* deemed legally incapable to make her own decision about accepting or refusing antibiotic treatment, we have to look backward in time to the most recent occasion when she did demonstrate legal capacity in relation to this issue.

When we make decisions according to this standard, the literature often refers to "privileging the wishes of the *then* person, that is, the "capable" person who wrote the directive over the *now* person, the "incapable one."

Mrs. Black, due to lack of legal capacity and autonomy, did not have her current wishes, interests, or values taken into consideration, though they are inferred by observers from her current actions, on the basis of standard folk

Dementia Ethics in a Hypercognitive Society," *Irish Journal of Psychological Medicine* 14, no. 4 (1997): 121–123.

psychological cues.[23] To me this approach is morally ham-fisted. It is as if Mrs. Black, by virtue of experiencing some psychological changes and the onset of some undeniable cognitive deficits, now has *no* wishes, interests, or values or, at least, none that matter.

Surely our default moral position ought to be that her values and interests *do* matter. We should not assume her arguable inability to frame her preferences and anti-preferences in terms of long-range plans, and intentions means that these things do not matter to her. And they ought to matter to everyone else concerned. Yet, the current working standard of autonomy requires us to cast our glances backward to the most recent prior capable expression of her wishes. It is the *former* Mrs. Black who is awarded status. In this case, it is her advance directive that identifies the values and interests that are supposed to matter today. Mrs. Black, as she exists now before our very eyes, fades to invisibility. An interesting phenomenon has just occurred. In all likelihood, the intent of all who care about her is to do "good" for her *currently*, so in that sense, the person who exists today matters very much. A while back, Mrs. Black wrote an advance directive to protect herself in the future from what she may have perceived as the ravages of dementia. She wrote her wishes back then based upon the values she had at that time. And she projected those values along with her wishes into the current time. But in another very real sense, she no longer currently matters in at least one very important way, as a human being who can continue to fashion for herself a life that matters to her *currently*. This is especially distressing for many of the staff who have known Mrs. Black across the continuum from mild to more severe dementia. They have witnessed the changes that her disease has brought, but overall they do not experience Mrs. Black to be all that different now from when they first came to know her. There is no distinct "pre-dementia" Mrs. Black for them to refer to. It is possibly as difficult for them to imagine her life as she experienced it prior to onset of her Alzheimer's Dementia just as it was most likely difficult for Mrs. Black to imagine a future life with dementia when she was fully capable and healthy. This is one reason why medical staff may be better situated to take Elysa Koppelman's advice, discussed later in this chapter—that we focus on the traits and gifts that a dementia patient has and not on those she has lost.

Remember what the point of autonomy is supposed to be outside of the pure narrow legal definition (where it is analogous to capacity) when we consider it from a practical point of view. Generally, it has to do with the right to make your own choices, to express your interests in ways that matter to you, or for that matter, in ways that are arbitrary and shortsighted should you so choose. Since Mrs. Black was not able to meet the legal criteria for autonomous/competent treatment decision-making with respect to her infection, there was the likely tendency that she would be viewed as generally incapable and nonautonomous. A dangerous leap has occurred. When the capacity card falls away, so to speak,

---

[23] Please recall the narrow, "hypercognitive," and "all or nothing" criteria that characterize these legal standards.

so does the one for autonomy. In practical terms, she is no longer currently allowed to make decisions for herself—at least the ones that others worry are not in her best interests. She has lost the right to make what the rest of the capable folks are allowed to make—potentially stupid decisions as well as smart ones.[24]

Some academics and ethicists go so far as to claim that our society has also created the problem of dementia in the first place, because of how we respond to the diagnosis and how badly we treat patients with dementia.[25] These writers object to an overemphasis on the idea that Alzheimer's reduces (or entirely destroys) who you are as a person, an idea that destroys in turn your status as *agent* whose preferences should be gleaned as much as possible and respected. Naturally, this approach has huge implications on how we understand patients' ability to make decisions or, at a minimum, to have decisions made for them that recognize their continuing to have and to demonstrate the values that are important to them.

The main emphasis we place on capacity in healthcare organizations is on answering the question of whether or not the patient is able to decide about specific medical treatment decisions. The legal and hospital administrative requirements drive this emphasis. The moral obligation, however, requires that we determine in what ways the patient is capacitated and how we will assist in enhancing and enabling these capacities. The conventional view that the patient has "lost" one's "self" and thus one's capacity as well is ill-conceived when it comes to persons with dementia. A more realistic and helpful approach is needed. I suggest we understand dementia patients as persons who are "whole" persons and are struggling to preserve their identities as much as possible. We become part of the caring community that plays a role in influencing how their sense of identity is experienced.[26]

(e) The Value of Values

Understanding autonomy (as legally construed in this domain) as mainly having to do with capacity in relation to medical decision-making can be very restrictive and unhelpful, when we try to apply the term to real-life healthcare scenarios. When I think about a richer and more "true to reality" idea of autonomy, I associate it with being able to express or live my life according to my values or ideals.[27] I do not know that I can provide a useful distinction between

---

[24] Generally speaking, we do not really worry about "smart" decisions incapable people make (which often means decisions incapable people make that cohere with what I, the professional, think is a "good" or "smart" decision) or "bad" decisions that are of very little consequence in terms of posing harm.

[25] See Stephen G. Post, 223–234; Tom Kitwood, *Dementia Reconsidered: The Person Comes First* (Buckingham: Open University Press, 2001), 7.

[26] Steven R. Sabat, "Capacity for Decision-Making in Alzheimer's Disease: Selfhood, Positioning and Semiotic People," *Australian and New Zealand Journal of Psychiatry* 39, no. 11–12 (Nov 2005): 1032; Tom Kitwood, *Dementia Reconsidered*, 103.

[27] As mentioned in an earlier note, Jaworska believes that well into the moderate stage of dementia patients can still retain the capacity to value and thus the capacity for autonomy. Surrogates can use

the terms of value, interest, and wishes. I imagine that "value" has a deeper meaning, perhaps more tied to my identity or sense of myself. It is perhaps more integrated into "who I am." My values are foundational to my interests and wishes, though I am uncertain as to how to distinguish a wish from an interest, other than to see interests as somewhat deeper than wishes.

Nonetheless, I do not think that from a practical, everyday-reality point of view, there is much use in trying to distinguish them from each other, for they overlap in many respects. For the purposes of trying to decide what to do from a moral point of view in terms of the issues confronting Mrs. Black, I do not wish to spend too much time deciding which one of the three terms is best to use. In this particular context, all three are interchangeable, more or less.

The values that are important to people significantly influence the decisions they make about current or future medical decision-making. Decisions are not made in isolation. They are often made in accordance with how they will affect loved ones and sometimes for the greater good of the public. People cite the desire to avoid being an emotional and financial burden on their children as a main motivator to writing advance directives that refuse treatment. Many people write directives because they do not wish to burden their loved ones with having to make painful end-of-life decisions for them. Some refuse medical technology resources such as expensive machinery that they feel others might have greater need for. Of course, decisions are also made out of fear of spending endless time attached to machines, perhaps prolonging a life of suffering. Some people worry that even when they are beyond suffering, a prolonged artificial life could be deeply undignified. They may not want to be kept borderline alive and "on display" in some undignified way for reasons partially overlapping with reasons why they wouldn't want their corpse to be subjected to indignities even after they are dead. Others worry that their family members or practitioners will make decisions for them that are not necessarily in their best interests and therefore wish to take matters "into their own hands."

When I reflect on the kinds of values that matter most to me, regardless of how enduring they have been or will prove to be in the future, the ways these values have been shaped have definitely been influenced by others. At the same time, I have also been a determining influence on the values that others hold. The influences on my values come from a variety of sources, well beyond the circle of my family and friends, but extend as well to other defining groups I am a member of, including my workplace, gender group, socioeconomic class, religious classification, North American culture, etc. Likewise, the options I am presented with by my healthcare team also reflect their values, as well as those that are supposed to underlie the laws, professional codes and practices of healthcare organization, and bodies to which the larger community is

---

the patients' existing values to help them translate them into specific medical decisions. She also believes that doctors have a duty to help enhance their dementia patients' capacity for autonomy. See Agnieszka Jaworska, "Respecting the Margins of Agency: Alzheimer's Patients and the Capacity to Value," Philosophy and Public Affairs 28, no. 2 (Spring 1999):110.

accountable. For example, note that the only treatment of choice offered in this situation was antibiotics. If, for example, I found myself to be in an institution that valued a more holistic approach to medicine, I (through my SDM) might also be offered naturopathic remedies. What I will be offered to choose from will reflect the values of the organization, and therefore, my freedom to express my values in terms of medical treatment decisions is influenced by the options made available to me. In this sense, it is partial or limited. But it is also partial in another important way, related to my ability to be a valuer, to hold values and to create new ones. Even some people with advanced Alzheimer's type should be recognized as having partial or limited autonomy, I hold, because they can still be valuers. Mrs. Black is a useful example of a valuer in the relevant sense, for reasons that bear detailing.

As we know, in the medical world, autonomy is understood as the (legal) capacity to make a treatment decision. This is all very well except for those patients with dementia that cannot demonstrate satisfaction of this legal requirement. When applied to people who lack this type of capacity, the autonomy standard is insensitive to the very real, if rationally disorganized, values they may possess. I have already referred to a larger sense of autonomy that is relevant to patients in the healthcare system and that has to do with the right to express oneself according to the values that matter most. The healthcare practitioners are concerned mainly with the specific decisions at hand. The decision is relevant for the patients too, of course, but only insofar as it coheres with their values. For example, Mrs. Black cannot, according to Ontario law, make an autonomous (or capable) post-dementia decision about accepting or refusing antibiotic treatment for her illness. However, she has certain values she seems to hold dear, ones that appear to give her life meaning, that provide her with a purpose to remain engaged and alive. And it seems to make every bit of sense to try to align medical treatment decisions with the values she seems to be expressing. The specific decisions made are not ends in themselves. They are the means by which the values get expressed.

I think of capacity not exclusively in terms of cognitive abilities to make medical treatment decisions one can understand and appreciate, but more broadly to include emotional, spiritual, religious, and social components. Mrs. Black might not be able to do the mental calculations involved in understanding all the technical terms a practitioner uses to explain a treatment-specific decision. Nor may she be deemed sufficiently able legally to appreciate the associated risks and consequences of the treatment, to a standard sufficient to the law. However, the areas of her brain responsible for storing emotional and social memories may indeed still fire and she still seems to value the feelings generated in her when family members (who she may not recognize) enter her hospital room.[28] She clearly enjoys that social experience. Even though she may not

---

[28] Jaworska refers to current findings in neurophysiology and in the neuropathology of Alzheimer's disease to defend the idea that valuing may be quite independent of grasping the narrative of one's life. The disease most severely affects the hippocampus, an area of the brain indispensable for

be in a position to draw or articulate the inference that she must remain living in order to continue to enjoy that experience, what matters is that this is true and that we recognize it. Respecting her continued status as an agent, albeit of diminished agency, requires us to work at gleaning her values, while recognizing her great vulnerability obliges us to intervene occasionally, to judiciously supply the instrumental reasoning and implementation of means to those values that she can no longer (reliably) herself contribute.

Many people with mild to moderate dementia (and perhaps even some with advanced dementia) may have desires, values, and interests that are important to them, even though they might not be able to consistently and clearly express them. Nonetheless, they are the context from within which medical treatment decisions ought to be made and preferably by the patients to the extent they are able. In many cases, others (family members, friends, or healthcare providers) who are most familiar with what the patients seem to value now can help determine which treatment decisions best fit. Nonetheless, there will always be some cases where this approach proves futile, and as a result, these patients' current wishes, interests, or values cannot be known with great confidence.

(f) How do we know which interests are more valued than others?

Much of the literature talks about there being two kinds of interests, "experiential" and "critical."[29] A further distinction can be made between interests and values.[30] The interests that are usually coined "critical" or "higher order" are often considered to be the kinds of interests that matter most. They are more highly valued than experiential interests. Critical interests are deeply pondered and long-standing, not mere whims of pleasure to be experienced in the here and now. They are very substantial and contribute significantly to a perpetual and stable identity. Unlike experiential interests, their value is independent of the immediate consequences that ensue. They tend to be translated into overarching goals related to the kind of life one chooses to live.

On the other hand, experiential interests are ones that we derive pleasure from in a more immediate sort of way. They are allegedly based on sensory pleasures, easily changed and fleeting. They tend to be more superficial, expe-

---

maintaining the sense of one's life as a whole, but not particularly important for the ability to value. Other areas of the brain are mainly responsible for reasoning and decision-making processes, particularly related to feelings and emotions and personal and social matters. A person's ability to value would be more likely to be compromised if these regions were damaged, which happens on an inconsistent basis and in more severe stages. She claims that some, but not all, of one's former values would likely be lost in the moderate stage. Jaworska, 121.

[29] Dworkin places higher value on critical interests, whereas Dresser prioritizes experiential interests; Jaworska, on the other hand, argues this distinction presents a false dichotomy. See Ronald Dworkin, *Life's Dominion: an Argument about Abortion, Euthanasia and Individual Freedom*, (New York: Alfred A. Knopf, 1993): 230; Rebecca Dresser, "Dworkin on Dementia: Elegant Theory, Questionable Policy," *Hastings Center Report* 25, no. 6 (1995): 36; and Jaworska, 108. Also some writers like Davis use the term "higher order "to connote critical interests. See J.K. Davis, "The Concept of Precedent Autonomy," *Bioethics* 16, no. 2 (April 2002): 132.

[30] It bears repeating that I think the distinction between interests and values is more blurred, as I think that values are really just interests we value. I use the terms interchangeably in this book.

rienced in the here and now more than considered with great reflection over the passage of time. Because of their immediacy, the short-term consequences associated with them count as valuable. For example, I may have a critical interest of living a life devoted to scholarship, continuing to challenge my own intellect throughout my life. This interest requires that I devote large amounts of time to my pursuit of academic stimulation. At the same time, I yearn to socialize with a chatty, humorous group of friends because it brings me immediate great pleasure. Yet doing so might threaten my devotion to the ongoing study.[31]

Who says one set of such interests is more superior than the other? And why can't my life be one that honors both, put into some sort of balance that seems to work for me? Perhaps I am the kind of person who prefers to live in the moment and trust my instincts more so than my reasoning when it comes to important decision-making.

One such expert in the field, John Davis, builds an argument that partly rests on the view that preferences that are more stable through time have more worth.[32] But many capable people express values and preferences that are not consistent over time. In fact, are we not supposed to be evolving through our lifetime, changing and growing in response to self-reflection? The more we self-reflect, the more our preferences and values might actually change. We do not necessarily have a defining set of values that remain constant throughout their lives.[33]

I think that values do change, can change, and in fact perhaps *should* change in response to altered life situations. In a sense, I think that changing one's values as a consequence of having different experiences might be a sign of one's capacity for self-determination (also known as autonomy). For example, we tend to look upon adolescence as a rite of passage where transformation of interests and values is supposed to be a positive sign.[34] It is reasonable to claim that the so-called loftier and deeper interests that are implicated in life being lived with an eye to its entirety can at the same time be the same ones that produce the most pleasure. So, perhaps it is not true to say that one type is better

---

[31] Wayne Shelton argues that we ought to respect experiential interests when critical interests are gone. He believes that critical interests of the "former self" are replaced by experiential interests as Alzheimer's disease progresses. Eventually, he espouses that experiential interests eventually disappear. At this point in time, the patient's prior critical interests and the preferences stated in the advance directive are to be given priority. Shelton, W (2016, January 7). Rethinking Dying and Alzheimer's Disease: How Do We Plan for Future Care? Retrieved from http://www.amc.edu/BioethicsBlog/post.cfm/rethinking-dying-and-alzheimer-s-disease-how-do-we-plan-for-future-care. Also see Paul T Menzel and Collette Chandler-Cramer, "Advance Directives, Dementia And Withholding Food And Water By Mouth," Hastings Center Report 44, no. 3 (2014): 23–37. They also confer that previous stated wishes of an advance directive should usurp waning experiential interests.

[32] J.K. Davis, 132.

[33] Dresser, *Dworkin on Dementia*, 35; Elysa R. Kopellman, "Dementia and Dignity: Towards a New Method of Surrogate Decision Making," *Journal of Medicine and Philosophy* 27, no. 1(2002): 80. In contrast, see Dworkin, 230.

[34] I thank Professor Tim Kenyon of Brock University, Canada, for this valuable insight.

than another, or that they can always be distinguished from each other, and with a difference that matters.

Another theorist, Agnieszka Jaworska, is correct to point out that the distinction between critical and experiential interests is a false dichotomy. It is possible for people with Alzheimer's dementia to value having certain experiences. She believes that people with dementia can have critical interests while the content base of them may be mostly experiential given their inclination to delight in simpler pleasures. "We cannot assume that a person with dementia has ceased to value just because he is now focused on his own pleasure and experience."[35] Even in the unlikely case that people with dementia can only have experiential interests, to say that only those persons who display critical interests count as having capacity (or the capacity for autonomy) is, in my opinion, built upon northing but "hypercognitive" ideology.

A number of theorists and ethicists have emphasized the importance of being able to grasp the narrative or "story" of one's life that is roughly understood to have continuity and semblance as a whole, in order for a person to remain a valuer.[36] Jaworska challenges this idea. I think that it is entirely plausible that persons without dementia have values or ideals that are deemed important to them in the present, independent of any explicit reference to the past or anticipated future life. That they can potentially think of those values in such diachronic terms is an important difference between them and persons with dementia. But should that make *all* the difference? It is important that we not raise the bar beyond what we would expect for persons without dementia and that we not construct sharp distinctions of autonomy between the two on arbitrary or vague grounds.[37] I think it is a myth to believe that most people make important decisions and/or hold onto significant values only within the context of an enduring life narrative. I doubt that some people would even be able to relate to the notion that there is some grand theme or narrative cohesion that ties all the parts of their lives somewhat neatly together. Even if it were to be the case that the concept of a narrative view coheres with most people's experience, and that Alzheimer's patients often lose the thread of their lives' narratives early on in the disease, it is too hasty to conclude that they are no longer able to value,

---

[35] Jaworska, 121.

[36] Mark G Kuczewski, "Commentary: Narrative View of Personal Identity and Substituted Judgment in Surrogate Decision Making," *The Journal of Law, Medicine & Ethics* 27, no.1 (Spring 1999): 33; Ben A. Rich, "Prospective Autonomy and Critical Interests: A Narrative Defense of the Moral Authority of Advance Directives," *Cambridge Quarterly of Healthcare Ethics* 6 (1997): 138.

[37] A number of theorists and ethicists advocate a lowering of the bar so that we do not inappropriately assess all people with dementia to be incapacity. See T. May, "Assessing Competency Without Judging Merit," *Journal of Clinical Ethics* 9, no. 3 (1998): 252; David C. Thomasma, "Beyond Autonomy to the Person Coping with the Illness," *Cambridge Quarterly of Healthcare Ethics* 4, no. 1 (Winter 1995): 12–22; J. Spike, "Narrative Unity and the Unraveling of Personal Identity: Dialysis, Dementia, Stroke and Advance Directives," *Journal of Clinical Ethics* 11, no. 4 (2000): 370.

or that their values ought not have some determinative role in their lives, just because they are now focused on immediate pleasures.[38]

From outside appearances, many patients with dementia appear to be living their lives moment-to-moment, caught up in the sensory experiences that confront them in the present. Others seem to inhabit the past more than the present. Possibly many live in both worlds. We presently cannot know whether patients with Alzheimer's dementia still have critical interests or, if they do, how enduring these are into the more severe disease stages. We cannot say with confidence that they are no longer able to hold onto the values they embraced in the past. Past values may remain currently relevant, but those suffering from Alzheimer's dementia often lack the instrumental means to express them. Nor can we know with any confidence that patients with dementia are incapable of forming new values applicable to their current lives.

Perhaps "abnormal" behaviors of persons with dementia can be understood to be meaningful expressions of their grief and despair, as they endure a sense of loss and try to hang onto what in the past has provided them with value and a sense of purpose. I suggest that it is the obligation of their loved ones and healthcare providers to assist these patients in holding onto the interests they seem to deeply value and derive meaning from, whether from the past or newly formed. Perhaps we should resist our tendency to pathologize behaviors that may not have immediate meaning to us but, nonetheless, have significance to those with Alzheimer's dementia.

One of the main reasons we make decisions in advance is because we care about what happens to us in the future, even if it turns out—and it may not—that we will be so cognitively impaired at that future time that we will not be able to care about ourselves or about those sorts of decisions. Even if many people with dementia are unable to form the kind of preferences that non-dementia people are (allegedly) easily capable of forming, why would we want to disqualify the preferences of the people with dementia as having no merit? Doing so is in great tension with the general aim of treating them with respect and dignity and has the effect of devaluing them as persons.

To summarize, I suggest we view Mrs. Black as partially autonomous and partially capable given that she seems to hold values that are important to her and is capable or able to express them to some extent. Additionally, there are others who can translate her values into action.[39] Despite her decreasing cognitive skills, she seems to be able to hold onto emotionally and socially based memories and possibly form some new ones. Nonetheless, the legal challenges remain. She does not seem able to sufficiently understand, in the pure cognitive sense, the information regarding acceptance or refusal of antibiotics for her infection, nor is she able to appreciate the consequences of such a decision. Nobody wishes to violate the law. Nor does it seem morally sound to apply a

---

[38] Jaworska, 121.

[39] Jaworska, 126.

legal standard whose criteria fail to capture the realities of dementia. This great divide is a perpetual source of moral distress in the healthcare workplace.

In addition, whether or not Mrs. Black's values or interests should be defined as critical or experiential is inconsequential. What matters is that she has them. When decisions patients make are related to interests of greatest importance, I think that capacity thresholds ought to be lowered in these situations. If the patient is unable to make a capable decision, SDMs ought to respect the current person's seeming values. At times, significant risks are associated with these decisions. It is commonplace thinking in healthcare contexts that one ought to be able to demonstrate greater capacity to make decisions which entail greater risks. What approach, then, ought to be taken given that one is incompatible with the other? I continue to uphold the argument in favor of lowering capacity thresholds. I will explain why.

At first blush, it seems intuitive to raise the capacity bar on decisions that could result in harm to the patient. But this does not square with the standard of autonomy, which also dictates that the reasons given for making decisions do not even have to be particularly sensible. Raising the capacity bar entails something like *really ensuring* that the patient understands the relevant information and can appreciate the risks, benefits, and consequences of the decision. Why this particular cognitive exercise, limited in scope as it is, should be considered essential, while at the same time evidence of (ir)rational thinking with regard to reasons underlying the chosen decision is inessential and irrelevant, is quite mysterious. Additionally, we ought to understand risk as being substantially subjectively determined. Perception of risk is person-sensitive, and thus it is unwise to evaluate it only against some general norm that means nothing to the patient considering treatment refusal options. Some people are by nature bigger risk takers, and thus they would be unfairly penalized if we were to up the ante so to speak, as far as the capacity required for this particular group of people. We are best not to interfere in terms of overriding or discounting another's wish, whether incapable or not, except for extreme situations when someone is not able to express any actions whatsoever from which values or interests might be gleaned, but rather to try to enhance the expression of the patient's wishes.

Additional Issues

Standards of Disclosure

The legal standard in Ontario upholds the "Reasonable Person" standard, which requires that the practitioner discloses the information that a "reasonable person in the same circumstances would require to make a decision about treatment."[40] I think

---

[40] See Ontario's *Health Care Consent Act*, 1996, s. 11 (2).

this standard is problematic. First, there are no definitions offered for the concepts of "reasonable person" as well as "same circumstances." The standard is vague and, as a result, I would venture it is either usually ignored or instead subjectively defined by the practitioners. Secondly, the term "reasonable" is supposed to apply to the general public. The information the practitioner discloses ought to be pertinent to what a hypothetical reasonable person needs in order to make an informed decision. But if the point of autonomy is to serve the wishes of the patient in accordance with *her* specific ways of being in the world, then it is misguided to think about anybody but her. When we consider the case of Mrs. Black, how would this standard help her physician to know what information she ought to impart to her? Is her reference point to be a reasonable patient who is "happy with dementia?"

From my experience at my workplaces, I think most practitioners tend to primarily use a professional practice standard when it comes to disclosure of information to their patients. The information they impart is largely determined by the particular professional community they identify with and usually conforms to the values and goals of that profession. The traditions of the particular workplace culture, coupled with the practitioner's own personal values, are influential as well. Earlier I mentioned that I often observe huge differences between practitioners in terms of what kind of information they share, the amount they impart, and the approaches they take. When I think more about this, I wonder if the great variance in part might be explained by attempts to customize this process according to the individual informational needs of their patients. As an ideal, the information that ought to be disclosed is the information that particular patient needs to have to make an informed decision *for her*. I admit it is very impractical, if not impossible, to expect that a practitioner would be so knowledgeable about their patients in so many realms of each of their lives that the practitioner could actually offer this kind of information. Nonetheless, I believe it is a standard we ought to prod practitioners toward. I think that some kinds of environments, such as long-term care environments, do lend themselves to the possibility that practitioners and patients can form long-range relationships that are shaped not just by the patients' medical needs but according to their values as well.

At a minimum, I suggest we adjust our explanations to patients according to what each would likely be able to understand and according to how they each might be best able to comprehend them. To whatever extent known, individual patient's wishes, values, and goals ought to some extent be determining of the information conferred. In Mrs. Black's case, the practitioner would need to try to explain the information as concretely as possible, with visual aids to help when necessary, such as showing her the medication, over a number of times if necessary, observing her responses, and trying to make meaning of them. Remember, the legal default position is to err on the side of assuming capacity, which in many cases will likely be partial anyway. What I am suggesting is unlikely to be implemented unless organizations are committed to providing sufficient educational and resource support for staff. From both a legal and moral point of view, staff must ensure they do everything possible to elicit understanding from each of their patients.

As aforementioned, in long-term care contexts, it is more likely that the practitioners have developed enduring relationships over significant periods of time with their patients. There are usually ample opportunities to learn from the patients, as well as from loved ones and other team members, which values seem currently to be the most highly held by each of their patients. If we think about the decision-making process as a collaborative effort taken on by the patients, the practitioners, and all others who know the patients best, then the kinds of information relevant to decision-making, as well as the best approaches to elicit the information, are likely to be revealed.

The main objective here is to be concerned with trying to enhance Mrs. Black's capacity rather than to ignore it. Ample time must be allowed for a thoughtful reflective process to occur, an idea that I also appreciate is often not well suited to the fast-paced and pressured environments that tend to exist in healthcare organizations.

The Context of Long-Term Care

Two of the three case studies I am presenting involve patients who are currently or have been in long-term care within healthcare settings. Many patients in long-term care have a diagnosis of dementia, as well as other chronic conditions.

Whether within the walls of a hospital or a nursing home, most patients spend years living within these environments. In that sense, they become their homes. The relationships formed with staff and volunteers are long term and are often described as close and very caring. In addition to forming fairly intimate bonds with the patients, staff members often develop significant degrees of familiarity with the families and friends of the patients. More often than not, the patients will die in these settings. Unlike an acute care setting, there is ample opportunity for the staff to interact with their patients on a frequent basis over a long period of time and to bear witness to the usual gradual decline of many cognitive and physical abilities. At the same time, they continue to develop relationships with patients who they get to know intimately and are often experts at understanding their body language, their grimaces, their gestures, and their moods, sometimes even to a greater extent than do family members and other loved ones. They often form deep emotional feelings of attachment and work very hard to ensure that their needs and wishes are complied with as much as possible.

These are environments where over time the patient usually requires greater dependence upon the staff, as is usually the case with patients with Alzheimer's disease. Mrs. Black relied more and more upon the staff to assist her with her hygiene, feeding, dressing, and decisional needs. The patients often rely on staff not only for their medical needs but also for their emotional and social needs. It is very moving to witness how knowledgeable a staff member can be about the intricacies of their patients' behaviors.

When working in such an environment, the legal concept of "autonomy" seems so alien, perhaps irrelevant, and maybe even inappropriate. The idea of patients making decisions completely *independently* is incongruent with the reality of aging and also with living with a dementia that increasingly incapacitates them as time goes on. Also the long-term care facility is a place of community where relationships matter greatly and where dependence upon others is the norm. The staff is there to assist the patients to live out the rest of their lives in ways that hold meaning for the patients for as long as is possible. The intent is to both understand and to help them to express whatever wishes—we could call this autonomy—and interests have meaning for the patients. It is thus important that loss of independence or "autonomy" is not construed in a negative way or else it will have devastating consequences on the self-esteem of the patients.[41] The focus should be on putting a positive value on dependence. It is reliance upon the support of others that is related to the idea of "relational autonomy"[42] where staff and loved ones "fill in the gaps" for the patients and also try to determine what is in each of the patient's best interests when doing so helps the patients realize the expression of their interests and values.

In Mrs. Black's case, her gradual decline makes it possible for staff and family to observe changes in her values or wishes over time. They will probably not be able to put their finger on the moment or the day that she became "so different." Again, the situation is somewhat different for the staff than it is for the family, as the former likely did not know Mrs. Black when she was completely free from the effects of her dementia. They have a different reference point than do the family members. Their involvement in the care of Mrs. Black is much more present oriented. They may not have "no other" Mrs. Black to compare her with or to be concerned about in terms of previous wishes. They cannot relate in the same way to a "previous Mrs. Black" to the same extent as can the family, who has had many more years relating to the pre-dementia Mrs. Black than to the current one. This also means they will probably not be mourning her loss (while she lives) in the same way her family members might. Nor would staff be privy to "capable" wishes in the same way as her loved ones would have. It is easy to see how different perspectives and relationship dynamics can render very different conclusions about the right thing to do.[43]

---

[41] See Daryl Pullman and Mark Kuczewski for more information. Daryl Pullman, "The Ethics of Autonomy and Dignity in Long-Term Care," *Canadian Journal on Aging* 18, no. 1 (1999): 26–46; Kuczewski, *Commentary: Narrative View*, 35. See Pullman for his explanation of how dignity as a concept instead of autonomy is more appropriate for long-term care facilities. Pullman, 34.

[42] For more information on the concept of "relational autonomy," see Elyssa Maeckelberghe, "Feminist Ethic of Care: a Third Alternative Approach," *Health Care Analysis* 12, no. 4 (Dec 2004): 317–327.

[43] I wish to emphasize that to be a member of the family or team does not necessarily preclude that all respective members share the same perspectives and/or conclusions about treatment decisions.

Is the Advance Directive Even Relevant?

I am not advocating in the case of Mrs. Black or others like her with partial autonomy that we completely ignore her advance directive. While I have tried to demonstrate the limitations of all advance directives in general, nonetheless, there might
be some role or purpose they might fulfill in current decision-making. I will examine this issue now. In part, I will address how we might approach the question about
the relevance of use of the advance directive.

Some theorists ask the question how we are to know if Mrs. Black's wish as
identified in her advance directive applies to her now.[44] I think this is a very appropriate question to ask but for different reasons than usually cited by others. The literature on the topic of advance directives usually conceptualizes the notions of
current "incapable" wishes and previous "capable" wishes (advance directives) as
being unrelated to each other and usually in conflict. Theorists and ethicists have
devised a whole range of arguments that lead to conclusions about why one ought
to take priority over the other. And it is from within this context that the question
raised above—how are we to know if there is coherence between her past and present wishes—draws its relevance. I argue that the context for this type of inquiry
should be based on how the advance directive can be used in a corroborative fashion, when it appears to cohere with current wishes. I do not intend to ask the question of whether we should privilege the directive or current wishes, as I believe we
ought, whenever possible, to try to honor current wishes over previous ones. The
directive can play a useful role in helping us understand more clearly what the
patient's current wishes are. Note the "directionality" differences between other
opinions and mine. They generally "start" with the advance directive. I start, and try
to end, with the current wishes and reflect backward primarily to clarify current
wishes.

John Davis, for example, is at considerable pains to establish how to determine
if a specific earlier wish remains a current one.[45] He does not provide direction
about what to do if a determination is made that the wish belongs to the past alone;
however, I am much less ambivalent. I believe that advance directives should not be
adhered to if they conflict with present wishes. However, advance directives may
give clues that can help explain what current wishes or values the patient is striving
to express. From my point of view of an ethicist, when the current wishes expressed
are perceived by SDMS to match those in the advance directive, it tends to have the
effect of increasing the confidence of SDMs, and team members, that they (the
SDMs) are making the right decision. This was the crucial element of coherence

---

[44] For example, see J.K. Davis, 114–133; David DeGrazia, "Advance Directives, Dementia and
'The Someone Else Problem'," in *Human Identity and Bioethics* (New York: Cambridge University
Press, 2005), 188.

[45] Professor Tim Kenyon rightly draws my attention to his idea that not only do we have difficulties
with confirming that a current wish coheres with a past one, we do not know ourselves as well as
we think we do, even when we express our thoughts and wishes when capable. The directionality
problem occurs both ways, both perspectively and prospectively. I thank him for this insight.

that I emphasized in discussing Mr. Black's case in Chap. 2. Family members often feel an enhanced sense of relief, and team members tend to experience much less moral distress under these decision-making circumstances.[46] Davis does, however, claim that if the current wish belongs to the past, we look upon it as a fresh exercise of autonomy and comply with it. Davis suggests an interesting, though not unproblematic, approach to determine if the current wish belongs to the past. He suggests we try to hypothesize what conversations would look like if the patients were asked if the reasons for their wishes in the directive are reasons that apply today. If they apply today, then their wishes are current and should be followed.

A number of problems arise. First of all, often the reasons underlying the wishes identified in an advance directive are often not known. Even if they were known, according to Davis, they only apply if they are based upon higher functioning interests, which in his opinion would also always be the most recent competent wishes.[47] We are to imagine what patients might say about their past reasons applying to all the current circumstances they are each in today, except that they would each have the capacity to understand this question and be able to competently respond.

Frankly, I find this approach unhelpful.[48] We are supposed to be imagining this scenario. This particular role entails a great deal of subjectivity and partly relies upon the person in this role having the requisite moral imagination to be able to fulfill the role of imagining this described situation.

---

[46] As a cautionary note, I added that I have witnessed some decision-makers go to extreme lengths to read into current behaviors of the patient with dementia in such a way that they make themselves believe there is coherence between the advance directive and what they perceive the current wishes to be. In these situations, they are committed to following the advance directive and will scramble to find corroborating "evidence" even when it does not seem to exist. Often, however, some family members or team members will raise objections, and the tendency to experience resultant moral distress is higher in these kinds of cases. The case study in the following chapter will reveal some of these challenges more concretely.

[47] J Davis, 131. As mentioned, I do not agree that we can distinguish types of interests in such a way and that it is a useful distinction to make even if we could. Even if we were to assume that the distinction is an important one, I challenge Davis's belief that the highest-order interests are also the most reflected upon and are always the most recent ones. He seems to be saying that there is a direct relationship between the amounts of time spent reflecting upon an interest and the value of that interest. I disagree. There are situations where that might happen to be true, but it is not necessarily always true. Perhaps a reflection of higher quality (whatever that means) requires less reflection time. Perhaps when I am fatigued, I require more time. Given that I disagree with Davis' criterion, as mentioned, it follows that I challenge his idea that the highest-order interests (again assuming for argument's sake that they exist) must be the most recent ones. Granted the most recent reflection has an advantage of breadth or scope in terms of numbers of past reflections it can consider. But how numbers translate into quality or benefit is still left unanswered. In any regard, if Davis is wrong (as I have tried to point out) about the highest-order interests being the longest ones reflected upon, it would not follow that the highest-order interests are necessarily the most recent ones. In addition, reflecting on all the past can change how we perceive an earlier preference. We can have a change of attitude or values and actually repossess a much earlier preference. If we readopt a former preference, while it might be temporally true that it is the most recent one, Davis would still need to prove that it is qualitatively the best one.

[48] In all fairness Davis does question whether or not what he is proposing is a sensible undertaking; however, he ends up giving it a fair amount of credibility. I, on the other hand, do not. Davis, 124.

Nonetheless, to Davis's credit, what distinguishes him from many other theorists is that at least he does not (initially) automatically disqualify persons with dementia from having current reasons or interests that ought to be considered. He accords them a certain status that others do not, others being ones who claim that if a person is incapable in the present with regard to a particular medical treatment decision, we ought to immediately look to the past capable person for most recent wishes. This latter approach basically ignores the person who currently has dementia, which Davis does not. However, in the end, he mistakenly concludes that Alzheimer's patients cannot have the kinds of interests that matter, and thus eventually he ends up in the same place as do other opinions I am critical of—that persons with Alzheimer's usually cannot be accorded the status of autonomy. Thus, unfortunately we would end up with privileging their advance directives exclusively, without considering at all the persons with dementia in front of us now.[49]

I suggest a modified approach. I would first look to the behavior that Mrs. Black exhibits, much like her healthcare team did. I would want to know what meaning Mrs. Black's behavior has for her in the context of her current life experiences.[50] What do her verbal and nonverbal behaviors say about her interests, values, and wishes? I would not be so concerned with the reasons behind the current wishes or previous wishes, but rather focus more on how to help her express her current ones. We need a context in order to decide whether or not the decision to accept or refuse a medical treatment coheres with her current wishes. I would want the staff and loved ones to collaborate in assisting her with expressing herself as much as possible. And, at the end of the day, all we will have is some stronger or not so strong hunches about what her current desires are. Her desires will not necessarily cohere with each other nor will we necessarily agree on the approach to take in order to take her perspective in assigning them priority. We will be hypothesizing about what we think her interests and wishes are, not claiming they can be known with any with certainty.[51] There are no specific approaches or answers that are absolutely correct. We will never know if the conclusion we reach was the best one because we can never know with certainty what Mrs. Black would have wanted at that particular time, or even know if she was confused herself and unsure about what she wanted, or could really know herself what she wanted. Part of the process entails the suspension of certainty. Being comfortable with "not knowing for sure" can be difficult for many people since trying to control the future is often what draws them to writing

---

[49] Pam Sailors offers another view worth considering. She suggests we consider the post-dementia person as a descendant of the pre-dementia person. The advance directive is not seen to be as authoritative as a regular will is. The descendant's best interests ought to be privileged. She views the relationship between the best interests and the advance directive as a mutually informing conversation. I concur with this idea and explain it further within this chapter. Pam R. Sailors, "Autonomy, Benevolence, and Alzheimer's Disease," Cambridge Quarterly of Healthcare Ethics 10 (2001): 190–193.

[50] Sabat and Post say similar things about the importance of meaning and context. See Steven R. Sabat, Capacity for Decision-Making, 1035; Stephen G. Post, Respectare, 223–234.

[51] Best to flirt with but never marry the hypothesis.

an advance directive in the first place. I imagine being in this scenario is quite counterintuitive to the mindsets of some, if not most, healthcare professionals.

I tend to agree with the staff that Mrs. Black's current behaviors demonstrate an interest in continuing to live the life she has now. This does not, however, preclude changes in her desire to do so at a future time. As mentioned, while my emphasis is on Mrs. Black's current wishes and values, I am not suggesting we necessarily disregard her interests in the past. First of all, I think it is illogical to think about ourselves as so distinctly divided by the passage of time and experiences and dementia illness. I think it is important to consider the whole person. Even in a more progressed stage of dementia, it seems counterintuitive to consider that a complete split has occurred in order to create what others like to conceptualize as the "then" person versus the "now" person.[52] Koppelman suggests that this sort of polarized thinking can seem more plausible than it ought to seem, if we focus on the deficits brought on by an illness and neglect the constant, persistent elements of the person. We should focus, argues Koppelman, on what remains of the self of Mrs. Black, not what has been lost, as well as what has shifted.[53] When I say "consider the whole person," I mean a more inclusive picture of the person over her life span and not just her cognitive functions but personality traits, religious views, spirituality, social desires, emotional characteristics, etc. Nonetheless, the bias I present is toward the person today, including her present experiences of herself in the state she is in now. We need to try to figure out what she is trying to convey through her behaviors, to attempt to understand the meaning of her current life as she is experiencing it, and it may or may not have much connection for her with her past. It is probably safe to assume that to the extent that we can determine or estimate that her values and wishes seem to be very different than they were before, then it is likely that her advance directive has little bearing currently. In any event, I cannot imagine it can have much weight even in the best case scenario, given all the problems that advance directives have in the first place. It might be of some use in a scenario where the person writes an advance directive targeted toward a temporary state of unconsciousness where upon afterward, the person is basically "returned" to their pre-unconscious state relatively unchanged.

Concluding Remarks

Let us return now to how we might continue to understand what to do, if anything, with Mrs. Black's advance directive. I would look to the advance directive not as the sole determinant in terms of what action to take, but rather as a particular tool. There is no value in choosing an approach that privileges the "then" person over the "now"

---

[52] Allen Buchanan and Dan Brock, Deciding for Others: The Ethics of Surrogate Decision Making, Cambridge: Cambridge University Press, 1989.

[53] Elysa R. Koppelman, "Dementia and Dignity: Towards a New Method of Surrogate Decision Making," *Journal of Medicine and Philosophy* 27, no. 1 (2002): 81.

person or vice versa. Both the autonomy and best interest standards have strengths and limits, so perhaps there is merit in using the advance directive to guide decision-making, but not in its usual way.[54]

Before I explore this idea more fully, let us review some important points. First of all, I have noted a number of problems that surround an advance directive: prediction problems, irreversibility, and both insufficient knowledge and insufficient appreciation of the pitfalls of having an advance directive. While some of these problems occur in everyday kinds of decision-making, there are particular degrees and types of problems that occur with advance directives that make them more problematic. Despite their limitations, I suggest we can still look to them not so much as an act of will that specifies what specific action to take, but rather as a piece of personal information that hopefully tells us something about Mrs. Black's values and wishes, as expressed at a certain time in a particular context. Clearly, we can tell from her advance directive that there were certain values that she was expressing. For me, one important question is similar to what Davis was getting at, and I state it as "what does Mrs. Black value about her existence today?" And when that question is pondered and responded to, by those in the best situation to draw inferences from her current behavior, then I would ask, "Is there anything in what Mrs. Black wrote in her advance directive that could help us better understand and appreciate her wishes and values now?" An advance directive might also prove useful when we are really in the dark about what a patient's values and best interests might be. A situation as such would probably be limited to very end stage dementia where the patient is close to being in a coma or near death.[55]

Prior to the very end, however, we have a person whose interests probably are either quite evident or potentially could be, if we take the time to get to know them as much as we can from this particular person's perspective of being in the world. This is a tall task undoubtedly, and not without its challenges, but it should be attempted. We start with the wishes we see being exhibited and look as well to this person's best interests.[56] This will be challenging because we then move into the subjective interpretation territory again and we know the limitations of such a world already. It is also perhaps an impossible task to calculate a balancing of risks and benefits because again these will be subjective in nature and also because there is a

---

[54] To reiterate, the principle of autonomy is usually associated with the "then" person as it is presumed that it was the "then" person who was capable to make an autonomous decision, such as that which is specified in an advance directive. The principle of best interest is seen as the "next best standard" and is applied when the patient is deemed incapable to make a treatment decision and there is no known prior capable wishes. Generally, this is the standard applied to decision-making for the currently incapable patient.

[55] L.K. Fellows, "Competency and Consent in Dementia," *Journal of the American Geriatrics Society* 46, no. 7 (1998): 926.

[56] Soren Holm reminds us that when interests conflict, we often are pulled to ascertain what is in someone's "best interest" as if there is just one trumping interest. Rarely is there only one. Soren Holm, "Autonomy, Authenticity, or Best Interest: Everyday Decision-Making and Persons with Dementia," *Medicine, Health Care and Philosophy* 4, no. 2 (2001): 153.

never-ending projection of consequences that will ensue in the future that are incalculable.

While from a legal point of view substitute decision-makers are the ones in Ontario to try to interpret advance directives, as I mentioned above, I think it makes sense to involve all relevant persons who are in the best position to know the patients currently, including perhaps those from the past who might add insight into the meaning of their advance directives from the context of when they were written. A popular suggestion from some noted theorists and ethicists regarding how to apply advance directives to current medical decision-making involves understanding that "people are their stories."[57] It reasonably follows that one's death is an essential part of one's story. However, I do not agree that it is the substitute decision-maker's role to ensure that the values embedded in the stories that the patient honored before should *necessarily* be the same ones that should be honored now. There is an assumption being made here, one that I believe to be mistaken, that implies continuance of values throughout one's life span. I have spoken earlier about the myth of this belief. Rather, it is up to those of us who can best help the patient to determine if it makes sense to apply a past value to a present situation automatically, when we have difficulties ascertaining what values are important to the patient now. I want to also reiterate at this point that we usually do not operate from a single value only, and there are all kinds of outcome possibilities that arise when we try to balance one value with another. Not only may we be inconsistent in our display of values, but even among those who hold the same value, a number of possible different decision outcomes could emerge. More than one option could arguably fit with someone's story.

Let us see how we might apply what I have written above to Mrs. Black's situation. Remember, she wrote that if she could no longer recognize her family members, she would not wish to receive treatment except to help with her pain reduction. I might argue that her recent pattern of current behavior, including attending the social programs, hugging everyone, and showing delight when anyone, including family members, enters her room, suggests she highly values relationships with others. Above all, this value seems central to her current existence. When I look back to her advance directive, I do not interpret her stipulation of loss of ability to recognize her family members as denoting loss of a value per se. I think the value she was upholding then is the same value she seems to be privileging now, which is her relationships with others. It is not the recognition per se that is of issue, at least according to my interpretation. Thus, I could conclude that the situation she identifies as being the trigger to withhold any treatment other than for pain does not currently exist. However, to be fair, I can imagine a different interpretation and conclusion being put forth, for example, that she was specific about recognition because she was speaking about the value of a certain level of capacity, not necessarily tying that in with the value of relationships. It is possible that what Mrs. Black meant was that she so valued her ability to be able to recognize her loved ones that

---

[57] See Kuczewski. He rightly includes Dworkin and Rich in agreement with this thought as well. Kuczewski, *Commentary: Narrative View*, 33.

if she lost that capability, she would want to refuse treatment. Interpretations about others' stories, and indeed even about our own, are highly subjective, and thus the conclusions that potentially will or can be drawn will vary considerably. The upcoming case of Mr. White in the next chapter is a great example of how two substitute decision-makers come to interpret their mother's current values and wishes very differently from each other. However, even if everyone shared the same interpretation, we are still left with the problem of what to do if current behavior seems to be indicating a value different than the one stipulated in the directive. Mrs. Black's son arguably is the one person who has known her the longest and is possibly the best person to interpret her directive, though we cannot assume that one follows from the other. And let us not forget that she has named him to be her attorney for personal care. That counts for a great deal, at least legally. Should his opinions, knowledge, and perspective not count as more valuable than those of the healthcare team?

I do not have a solution to the problem of what to do in the face of different interpretations and different conclusions as noted above. There have been a variety of suggestions put forth, including one where substitute decision-makers are to imagine a discussion occurring now between themselves and the former capable persons who wrote the advance directives, where the substitute decision-makers are in the role of helping the current patients express their values.[58] In this scenario, the son is to keep the current Mrs. Black in mind while imagining a conversation with his mother at the time she wrote the advance directive. A variation of this idea is put forth by Kuczewski.[59] He suggests that the son should imagine having such a discussion with his mother, but not at the time she wrote the directive. Instead, he should focus on what his mother might reveal about her values today if she could express herself succinctly in the present. I am not sure that one variation is better than another, partly because I know of no objective standard to use to measure such imaginings, and I certainly have no way of knowing whether substitute decision-makers are doing what the law requires of them, even if they wanted to assume that role. For example, it is unclear how this would address the hopefully very rarely occurring worry, if it otherwise a reasonable one, that the son only wants his mother to die sooner than later because perhaps he stands to inherit a few million dollars or can no longer tolerate his visits with her or the guilt that he experiences as a result of not visiting her.

---

[58] See Blustein who talks about the substitute decision-makers trying to put themselves in the role of continuers of the views of the persons who wrote the advance directives. Jeffrey Blustein, "Choosing for Others as Continuing a Life Story: the Problem of Personal Identity Revisited," *The Journal of Law, Medicine and Ethics* 27, no. 1 (1999): 20. Another variation on this theme is to see the advance directive not as an exercise of autonomy in the sense of a wish to be followed regardless of consequences, but rather as something that resembles the values of the best interest standard. See Penney Lewis, "Medical Treatment of Dementia Patients at the End of Life: Can the Law Accommodate the Personal Identity and Welfare Problems?" *European Journal of Health Law* 13, no. 3 (2006): 231–234; and Anthony Wrigley, "Personal Identity, Autonomy and Advance Statements," *Journal of Applied Philosophy* 24, no. 4 (2007): 382.

[59] Kuczewski, *Commentary: Narrative View*, 33.

Regardless of what version might be preferred, and there are of course other options not considered here that could potentially be worthy of consideration as well, we are always left with subjectively interpreting the meaning of the contents of the advance directives and subjectively interpreting the meaning of the current patients' behaviors. Nothing we can do can eliminate the interpretative aspect. Regardless of how close the substitute decision-makers are/were to the patients, there is no standard by which to measure the accuracy of subjective interpretation, nor is there a conclusively superior reference point. Similar to our challenge of not knowing how to improve upon the "appreciation" problem of informed consent, we are left wanting to ensure our subjective interpretations of others' advance directives coheres enough with what the authors intended to convey. Yet, we cannot really know if there is alliance as such. In the same vein, we assign meanings to current behaviors of patients with dementia in order to try to ascertain what their present wishes are. We can, of course, speculate, but not really know them.

My experience shows me again and again that there are often numerous and varying interpretations and meanings that can be assigned to the same observed behaviors.[60] However, we usually have a variety of opportunities to attempt to understand what is being communicated to us currently and can continue to observe patients over a number of instances. A second advantage is that current interpretation of current behaviors can be shared with and evaluated against those of other current reliable witnesses and observers.

I reiterate that we have in front of us Mrs. Black, who should be deemed to be partially autonomous on the basis of being a valuer. It would make sense to "figure out how her values would be best upheld in a reality she no longer fully understands, as well as helping her implement these solutions in practice."[61] Even by the legal standard where she would likely be deemed to be incapable, we would have an obligation to "consider incapable wishes" as part of a best interest standard. However, from a legal point of view, we would only consider this standard if she were incapable to consent to treatment currently, *and* we did not know her previous capable wishes that would be applicable to the current situation.

I am advocating that her previous capable wishes are not binding on the current situation, because she was not sufficiently informed to make an autonomous choice.[62] I therefore think it is a serious mistake to consider her wishes *then* as her

---

[60] And, I add, both across various observers and also forthcoming from the same observer.

[61] Jaworska, 134.

[62] However, at one earlier point in time, I wondered if it would be reasonable to consider Mrs. Black's advance directive as minimally or partially autonomous (as happens to be what we consider her current wishes to be) because of all the flaws I have earlier discussed. Doing so might render it competitive with her current wishes and bring us right back to our initial question of whether to privilege her current wishes or those of her advance directive. However, current expressions of values and interests (also known as current autonomy) are supposed to trump former expressions of values and interests (precedent autonomy) so we would still end up privileging her current wishes. Due to the limitations referred to with regard to Mrs. Black's advance directive, I already established that it would be reasonable to consider her directive to be more like a past wish that she expressed without undue significance. However, I can envision a potential scenario where

capable wishes *now* as a legal standard of (precedent) autonomy. I agree with the position claims of others who suggest we should not apply a standard of "autonomy" to advance directives. This change would ultimately lower the status of advance directives and legitimize their use much less frequently. The directives could qualify as interests or wishes stated in the past, with no special privilege over and above the interests or wishes that are being expressed today. If these past wishes cohere with current interests or wishes, then they could potentially serve to make the substitute decision-makers or healthcare professionals more confident about decisions being made in the present. I suggest that if they do not, then they are of very little relevance in the present.

In my thinking, a best interest's standard is a better fit with the notion of the whole person. This standard takes into account both past and present values and wishes. A calculation is undertaken of all these interests in terms of risks and benefits for the patient presently, as well as with a view to the future. Unlike the autonomy standard that concerns itself with current interests of the patient only when the patient is deemed capable to the treatment decision at hand, the best interest standard in part considers the current wishes of the patient with dementia.

Given the altered notion of autonomy that I am suggesting, which includes the possibility of it being partial and relational,[63] there is room for both autonomy and best interests. I want to also emphasize that perhaps we ought not to consider them so separate anyway. Remember that autonomy has to do with the notion that the individual person is the best one to decide which interests one wants to make one's own and that it is best that others not override them. With the notion of relational autonomy, we need others to help determine what those interests might be from the perspective of each patient in situations where they cannot express them in ways readily understood. We might need to assist the patients in carrying them out if they are unable to do so; however, this does not mean that the patients no longer have interests. We are not to substitute ours for theirs! While we will be keeping an eye out for Mrs. Black's best interests from her perspective, we can never know them for sure. A risk of trying to get as close to her view as possible is that we end up confusing our views for her views as we project what we think, mistaking them for hers.

---

an advance directive might be useful. That might be when someone is in a situation where for all intents and purposes the person does not have any current active interests or values as an agent (perhaps being in a coma could qualify), and had previously written an advance directive about what treatment was to be refused, in anticipation of a future coma. Granted, this person would not be able to appreciate what that comatose experience would be like, or how it would be subjectively experienced, so we have the same prediction problems as usual. However, while being in a coma, the patient would not then experience oneself to have interests or values, so precedent autonomy or most recent previous wishes would not be in conflict with any future ones since there would be no future ones to be in conflict with, at least that the patient would be experiencing. The person could still of course have interests that matter, such as being treated with dignity, etc., but as far as we know regarding comas, the patient would not be experiencing them. The advance directive would really be tantamount, I suppose, to the regular kind of wills that are written with the anticipation of future death.

[63] See Chap. 1 footnote no. 22 for initial reference to "relational autonomy."

I happen to be an ethicist who privileges the current wishes, partially autono-mous, partially capable as they may be. In the case of Mrs. Black, so did all the members of the healthcare team. However, maybe I was projecting my own values and interests onto Mrs. Black. I do not know this. I do think that if I was seemingly living happily with dementia, I would want to continue to live. But perhaps I am as guilty as is everyone else who also uses their imagination to project into the future. Short of actually being in that experience, I cannot really know now what I may want later. Perhaps everyone else on the team may have been projecting their own personal values of wanting to keep Mrs. Black alive. We cannot know this for sure. However, as stated earlier, I think it is always good practice to try to make transpar-ent for ourselves and for others the interests and values that are influencing our own opinions and recommendations.

What if someone on the team considered Mrs. Black's current wishes, but decided to give more weight to the wishes she expressed prior to the onset of her dementia? This seems to be what her son in fact did. There is no objective reason either to disqualify his preference or to affirm it. By definition, anyone's identified interest is of value and of relevance. It is not possible to assign a quantitative figure to any one particular interest. However, perhaps we could stipulate that the calcula-tions ought to produce a net interest result that favors the current values and wishes, whenever possible over the past ones, if they conflict. A reasonable rebuttal, how-ever, could be that if we are going to end up privileging her current wishes, why should we be bothered with such calculations in the first place? Just declare the most recent wishes as the default standard in the first place. I think we can fairly safely presume that the wishes of most Alzheimer's patients would not be premised upon contemplation of a future. Perhaps it would be reasonable to override current wishes when consideration of each patient's best overall interests, entailing both the present and the future, renders their current wishes harmful.

However difficult the use of this standard might prove to be, in its traditional form or as modified by me as suggested above, it is still morally superior in my view because it takes into account the current experiences of persons with dementia as living human beings of worth. While the adaptation of this standard to everyday medical treatment decision-making relating to patients with dementia is very chal-lenging, it nonetheless holds heightened moral promise. We can understand Mrs. Black's display of delight over social interactions to be either an interest or an expression of autonomy—partial or minimal—or possibly both. I suggest that the borders between these two standards start to disappear when we admit that capacity to make decisions can be partial and that patients with dementia can be able to hold values right up to the end of their lives in some situations, regardless of whether they rely on others to supply the means of action. The challenge is to move away from the theoretical vagueness and generalities of legal terms, and try to apply interests and wishes that make sense for the current patients in their current experiences, with an eye to the consequences for them in the future. When we cannot feel very confi-dent, we must work very hard until we can glean some meaning about their held values from their behaviors or until we are utterly convinced that we cannot.

Mrs. Black's current wishes generally take precedence over her former ones, just like they do with anybody else who is not considered incapable. In this case, there is an additional important consideration to take into account. Unless there is general belief that a patient is suffering to an extent that is too excessive (and again this involves subjective interpretation), healthcare providers are usually more morally comfortable with deciding on the side of extending life. And I think this is right mainly because not to do so carries greater risks that individual practitioners' views alone will determine whose life is morally worthy of being saved. And, as mentioned before, those in the business of delivering healthcare generally try to save lives.

In the case of Mrs. Black, the physician in need of consent in order to administer the treatment accepted the refusal from the son based upon the advance directive. Why? We know that he felt that withholding of treatment would be going against both her current wishes and interests, which he believed mattered greatly. Furthermore, he was completely aware of how much the son's decision would factor in contributing to significant moral distress for him and his teammates. Since the son was named the legal attorney for personal care for Mrs. Black's personal care, which includes medical treatment decisions, he not only has the legal power to make decisions according to her wishes in the advance directive, he has the obligation to do so if she is currently incapable and her previous wishes apply to the present circumstances. The physician would need to go before a legislated board to challenge the son's decision. The reality was that this physician did not want to venture into a conflict with the SDM, nor did anyone else on the team wish to initiate such a potentially divisive process.

What if the son had argued that his mother's advance directive should not be followed, because she demonstrates such happiness at this time and she could not have predicted that she could live so happily with dementia, and thus her directive cannot be applied to the current circumstances? Or, he may have argued that we should privilege her best interests over her (precedent) autonomy just because it makes more common sense to do so. He may ask a very relevant question: "Why should autonomy always trump best interests anyway?" Who is to say that there aren't other reasons, aside from autonomy, to keep her alive?[64]

In this scenario, Mrs. Black's son would have been in agreement with the team and likely no one would have challenged the fact that her advance directive was not being followed. She would have received the treatment. Everyone would have been happy. I have argued in this chapter that likely Mrs. Black was capable of partial autonomy. However, in the event that she was not, I would still agree with the healthcare team that the best interest standard *should* be used as the justification to administer medication to her as the default standard. According to current law, however, this would not be appropriate to do as the law recognizes autonomy as the default standard.

---

[64] Newton, 19. Let us assume for the moment that he believes that his mother is not even "partially autonomous" and he is referring to the legal standard of best interest.

Let us remember, however, that Mrs. Black's son was not in agreement with the team and a decision needed to be made. There were two distinct camps operating. Her son read her words literally and as being definitive. He did not consider the option of overriding the directive; however, the team was united in their view that the advance directive ought to be overridden so that Mrs. Black's current wishes could be honored instead. Neither camp was willing to change its position. Sometimes, as shown in the first case of Mr. Black, there just happens to be a consensus between all the players. But the fact that there was coherence between the healthcare team members and family members did not necessarily mean there was coherence with the wishes of the person with dementia, because we could not really know what Mr. Black wanted currently. Kuczewski holds that "more likely advance directives make healthcare providers more confident about choices made, not surrogates."[65] This was untrue in the case of Mrs. Black, whose case is not obviously rare or idiosyncratic. Nonetheless, healthcare providers often recognize how difficult decision-making for their patients with dementia is, and often appreciate the fact that substitute decision-makers will make these kinds of tough calls. This does not mean that they necessarily agree with the decisions made at all times, nor does it mean that we can know with great confidence that we have met the best interests of the patients and/or made decisions that were in line with their current values. Nonetheless, in the case of Mrs. Black, our entire team believed that we failed her on both counts.

In the next chapter, I will take a closer look at what the literature has to say about the substitute decision-makers' role, and whether or not SDMs actually do make decisions according to the legal standards they are supposed to follow. Remember, regardless of what standards they do or do not use, their conclusions are highly interpretative and subjective. This raises the important question about how close anyone can ever really come to knowing what is in the best interest of another.[66]

Sources

Beauchamp, T.I., and J.F. Childress. *Principles of Biomedical Ethics*. New York: Oxford University Press, 2001.

Blustein, Jeffrey. "Choosing for Others as Continuing a Life Story: The Problem of Personal Identity Revisited." *The Journal of Law, Medicine and Ethics* 27, no. 1 (1999): 20–31.

Buchanan, Allen and Brock, Dan. *Deciding for Others: The Ethics of Surrogate Decision Making*. Cambridge: Cambridge University Press, 1989.

Davis, J.K. "The Concept of Precedent Autonomy." *Bioethics* 16, no. 2 (April 2002): 114–133.

DeGrazia, David. "Advance Directives, Dementia, and 'The Someone Else Problem.'" *Bioethics* 13, no. 5 (1999): 373–391.

Dresser, Rebecca. "Advance Directives in Dementia Research: Promoting Autonomy and Protecting Subjects." *IRB: Ethics and Human Research* 23, no. 1 (Jan–Feb 2001): 1–6.

---

[65] Kuczewski, *Commentary: Narrative View*, 34.

[66] See Welie re: "moral strangers". J.V. Welie, "Living Wills and Substituted Judgements: a Critical Analysis," *Medicine, Health Care and Philosophy* 4, no. 2 (2001): 171.

Dresser, Rebecca. "Dworkin on Dementia: Elegant Theory, Questionable Policy." *Hastings Center Report* 25, no. 6 (Nov–Dec 1995): 32–38.

Dworkin, Ronald. *Life's Dominion: An Argument about Abortion, Euthanasia, and Individual Freedom*. New York: Alfred A. Knopf, 1993.

Fellows, L.K. "Competency and Consent in Dementia." *Journal of the American Geriatrics Society* 46, no. 7 (1998): 922–926.

Firlik, Andrew. "A Piece of My Mind: Margo's Logic." *Journal of the American Medical Association* no. 265(1991): 191.

Gather, Jakoy and Vollmann, Jochem. "How to Decide?Evaluating the Will of a Person with Dementia in the Light of Current Behavior, Advance Directive and Legal Representatives' Perspectives", *GeoPsych* 28, no. 1 (2015): 17–20.

Health Care (Consent) and Care Facility (Admission) Act, R.S.B.C. Health Care (Consent) and Care Facility (Admission) Act, R.S.B.C. 1996, c.

Holm, Søren. "Autonomy, Authenticity, or Best interest: Everyday Decision-Making and Persons with Dementia." *Medicine, Health Care & Philosophy* 4, no. 2 (2001): 153–159.

Jaworska, Agnieszka. "Respecting the Margins of Agency: Alzheimer's Patients and the Capacity to Value." *Philosophy and Public Affairs* 28, vol. 2 (Spring 1999): 105–138.

Koppelman, Elysa R. "Dementia and Dignity: Towards a New Method of Surrogate Decision Making." *Journal of Medicine and Philosophy: A Forum for Bioethics and Philosophy of Medicine* 27, no. 1 (2002): 65–85.

Kuczewski, Mark G. "Commentary: Narrative View of Personal Identity and Substituted Judgment in Surrogate Decision Making." *The Journal of Law, Medicine & Ethics* 27, no. 1 (Spring 1999): 32–36.

Lewis, Penney. "Medical Treatment of Dementia Patients at the End of Life: Can the Law Accommodate the Personal Identity and Welfare Problems?" *European Journal of Health Law* 13, no. 3 (2006): 219–234

Maeckelberghe, Elyssa. "Feminist Ethic of Care: A Third Alternative Approach." *Health Care Analysis* 12, no. 4 (December 2004): 317–327.

May, T. "Assessing Competency Without Judging Merit." *Journal of Clinical Ethics* 9, no. 3 (1998): 247–257.

Menzel, Paul T and Chandler-Cramer, Collette. "Advance Directives, Dementia And Withholding Food And Water By Mouth." *Hastings Center Report* 44, no. 3 (2014): 23–37.

Newton, Michael J. "Precedent Autonomy: Life-Sustaining Intervention and the Demented Patient." *Cambridge Quarterly of Healthcare Ethics* 8, no. 2 (April 1999): 189–199.

O'Neill, Desmond. "Cogito Ergo Sum? – Refocusing Dementia Ethics in a Hypercognitive Society." *Irish Journal of Psychological Medicine* 14, no. 4 (1997): 121–123.

Post, Stephen G. "*Respectare*: Moral Respect for the Lives of the Deeply Forgetful." In *Dementia: Mind, Meaning, and the Person*, edited by Julian C. Hughes, Stephen J. Louw and Steven R. Sabat, 223–234. Oxford: Oxford University Press, 2006.

Pullman, Daryl. "The Ethics of Autonomy and Dignity in Long-Term Care." *Canadian Journal on Aging* 18, no. 1 (1999): 26–46.

Rich, Ben A. "Prospective Autonomy and Critical Interests: A Narrative Defense of the Moral Authority of Advance Directives." *Cambridge Quarterly of Healthcare Ethics* 6 (1997): 138–147.

Sabat, Steven R. "Capacity for Decision-Making in Alzheimer's Disease: Selfhood, Positioning and Semiotic People." *Australian and New Zealand Journal of Psychiatry* 39, no. 11–12 (November 2005): 1030–1035.

Sailors, Pam R. "Autonomy, Benevolence, and Alzheimer's Disease." *Cambridge Quarterly of Healthcare Ethics* 10 (2001): 184–193.

Schermer, Maartje. "In search of 'the good life' for demented elderly." *Medicine, Health Care and Philosophy* 6 (2003): 35–44.

Shelton, Wayne. "Rethinking Dying and Alzheimer's Disease: How Do We Plan for Future Care?" (January 7, 2016). Retrieved from http://www.amc.edu/BioethicsBlog/post.cfm/rethinking-dying-and-alzheimer-s-disease-how-do-we-plan-for-future-care.

Spike, J. "Narrative Unity and the Unraveling of Personal Identity: Dialysis, Dementia, Stroke and Advance Directives." *Journal of Clinical Ethics* 11, no. 4 (2000): 367–72.

Thomasma, David C. "Beyond Autonomy to the Person Coping With Illness." *Cambridge Quarterly of Healthcare Ethics* 4, no. 1 (Winter 1995): 12–22.

Welie, J.V. "Living Wills and Substituted Judgments: a Critical Analysis." *Medicine, Health Care & Philosophy* 4, no. 2 (2001): 169–183.

Wrigley, Anthony. "Personal Identity, Autonomy and Advance Statements." *Journal of Applied Philosophy* 24, no. 4 (2007): 381–396.

Chapter 4
Mr. White

Mr. White

Mr. White is a 62-year-old gentleman, widowed, with three grown children, the eldest being a daughter, Jamie, who has lived in a government-sponsored residence for persons with severe intellectual deficits, for most of her life, and twin children, a son, Alex, and a daughter, Brie, both married. Mr. White had been enjoying an active, healthy, and fulfilling life, filled with close family and friends, frequent travel, and a successful career as a chef. Approximately 2 years ago, his friends noticed that he was experiencing memory loss beyond what is usually attributed to normal aging. After nearly burning his house down because he left a pot of water boiling on the stove for a few hours, he agreed to be assessed at a reputable outpatient memory clinic. Results yielded a diagnosis of mild stage Alzheimer's dementia.

Frightened and distressed, Mr. White tried hard to continue to lead his usual life. Nonetheless, he was becoming increasingly confused and anxious about how to manage his catering contracts and, subsequently, lost some good clients. After another safety mishap at home, coupled with a significant decline in his finances, he reluctantly agreed to sell his business and move in with his son, Alex, and his daughter-in-law, Beverly. While initially it proved to be a challenging adjustment for the three of them, eventually they all settled into their new living arrangement. Alex and Beverly were very caring and supportive of Mr. White. His daughter, Brie, who lived nearby, visited very regularly, often playing the piano for her father, an activity he looked forward to with great enthusiasm.

One and a half years later, Beverly gave birth to a premature son. Given both the needs of the new parents to tend to their frail infant and the increasing memory loss and associated frustration and moodiness of their father, Alex and Beverly felt they had no choice but to suggest alternative living arrangements for him. Mr. White was outraged, denied increased coping problems, and in fact saw himself as a potential babysitter to his new grandson. While his son and daughter-in-law empathized with him and wished they could accommodate his desires, they worried about his lack of

© Springer International Publishing AG 2018
M. Sokolowski, *Dementia and the Advance Directive*,
https://doi.org/10.1007/978-3-319-72083-8_4

insight into his own difficulties and felt that they had no choice but to strongly encourage him to move into a nursing home. Mr. White pursued the option of living with his other child, but Brie's husband, Lance, opposed the idea as their small apartment would not afford them much privacy. Additionally, the couple was contemplating a move to another country as a result of an alluring job offer. As a result, a search for an appropriate long-term care placement was undertaken.

Six months later, a desirable spot became available, and Mr. White's family helped him move onto a floor that houses residents with dementia. Mr. White found the transition to long-term care residence to be very challenging. He felt like a misfit, being at least a decade or two younger than the majority of his fellow residents. He was angry that he was burdened with "the death sentence of Alzheimer's" at such a young age. He also began to experience frequent headaches and nausea. He desperately missed his independence and the reputation he had enjoyed only 2 years earlier as a talented chef. One of the facility's consulting psychiatrists diagnosed him with depression. Mr. White agreed to take antidepressant medication, which helped him considerably. He also received a drug that was known to be successful in slowing down the progression of Alzheimer's disease. Gradually, Mr. White became less depressed and began to participate in the social and recreational programs offered.

Two months later, Mr. White received additional distressing news confirming a diagnosis of an inoperable brain tumor. He was given a prognosis of about 9–12 months to live. Understandably, he and his children were devastated. Initially, Mr. White seemed to comprehend the information he received. However, over the ensuing few days, occasional bouts of memory loss and confusion were noted. At times, he would be found wandering the halls late at night, disoriented and confused as to where he was. When asked what he understood about Alzheimer's disease, he stated it was related to memory loss but attributed this to an allergy he had. His experiences of confusion were expected to increase as his tumor grew. During the next week, he occasionally asked his children and staff members to remind him of the name of the "new" disease he had. He seemed to be easily reminded. When asked what he remembered about being told about the tumor, he said, "I will die from a terrible death soon. My disease will eat away at my body and my brain." Unfortunately, Mr. White's speech was beginning to slur at times, and his headaches occurred more frequently. One week later, Mr. White's twin children spoke to their father in order to elicit his agreement to meet with a lawyer to review and/or update his legal will. They believed their father understood their request and thought it was a good idea. In fact, they learned from a nurse on his team that he had mentioned the idea to her and indicated it was a good idea. Mr. White was able to state that he thought about doing this a while ago and was happy to talk about his treatment wishes with his lawyer as well. A few days later, his lawyer, a gentleman he knew for a number of years, met alone with him. At that meeting an advance directive for personal care was also drawn up, naming the Mr. White's twins jointly as attorneys for personal care.

Mr. White's physical condition rapidly deteriorated over the next few weeks. He had tremendous difficulty enunciating his words. Often, he was short of breath and tended to choke when he ate or drank. His motor skills were declining fairly rapidly, and he had tremendous difficulty with writing at this point, in order to communicate. Generally, he was tearful and frustrated.

The team felt the urgency of his rapid decline. They worried that advancing neurological and cognitive decline would soon render him incapable to express his treatment wishes. They arranged a meeting with him and his twin children (with Mr. White's permission) in order to try to derive directions from him about the near future medical treatment decisions he would likely be asked to make.[1] The physician next explained that, within a week or 2, he would probably no longer be able to take food and water by mouth. To be kept alive, he would need a feeding tube inserted into his abdomen. He gave him basic information related to the tube, reviewed its potential benefits as well as risks, and asked for his consent to receive it. He shook his head, indicating "no." Being aware of his difficulties in expressing himself, his physician and respective team members were uncertain if he was able to understand and appreciate the consequences of his refusal. Perhaps he was but was unable to communicate effectively to them. Mr. White's son produced his advance directive and asked him if those wishes were reflective of his current wishes as well. He reviewed its content, which made reference to his wishes to "die with dignity," to "receive any and all pain medications offered to reduce or eliminate any suffering he might experience," and to "have no heroic measures" attempted. Tearfully, he nodded his head in agreement throughout the reading. Other staff members asked him to clarify what he meant by the terms, "no heroic measures" and "death with dignity." Mr. White tried to speak, but could not be understood. When asked if he still wanted what he wrote in his advance directive, he nodded "yes." He repeated the same response, two or three times again, when the same question was repeated. He was again asked a couple more times if he wanted a feeding tube, and consistently shook his head, indicating "no." When asked if he had any questions about the feeding tube, he nodded, "yes." However, despite several attempts, he was unable to enunciate the words well enough to be understood. He became very angry and frustrated and indicated he wanted to go back to his room. He was clearly exhausted. He was reminded that he had more time to consider what he wanted. When the physician asked his permission to continue to meet with us in his absence, he nodded in agreement.

The meeting continued. Brie believed that the new diagnosis was very hard for her father to accept, and that he was understandably traumatized by all the bad news, and therefore not in any frame of mind to make a rational decision at this moment. Brie stated that it would be "wrong" not to give her father a feeding tube. She was certain that her father was "not ready to die" and therefore would accept the treatment but needed some time.

When asked what she thought about her father's advance directive, Brie replied that the lawyer had probably rushed him through the process, and, as a result, he was forced to complete it without much thought (the nurse had noted in the chart that the

---

[1] As we know, the full force of an advance directive only comes into play if the patient is no longer deemed competent to either refuse or accept a specific medical treatment.

lawyer was present for 20 min). Brie surmised that probably the advance directive did not *necessarily* represent what her father would want. She expressed uncertainty about what her father meant by the words "dying with dignity," and "no heroic measures." She described her father as generally a very strong, independent man who more recently turned to her and her brother for decision-making support since his diagnosis of Alzheimer's disease. Alex noted that the roles in their family had since become reversed. He and Brie seemed more like parents to their father than the other way around. He noted aloud that their father underwent a similar personality change 10 years ago, when their mother unexpectedly died. Slowly over time, however, he became "more like his old self" until the diagnosis of Alzheimer's, at which time he seemed to revert back to feeling more emotionally fragile.

Alex disagreed that his father would want a feeding tube. He understood his refusal to be consistent with his rejection of any heroic measures. He claimed that, since his diagnosis of the brain tumor, on many occasions he had told him that he did not want to continue living. His eyes blinked away tears as he recalled how he pleaded with him to help him kill himself. "Look," he said emphatically. "He does not want to live his last few precious months attached to tubes. Give him pain medication as he stated in his directive, and let him be. He does not want a feeding tube!"

The physician stated he first had to determine if Mr. White was currently capable to express his wishes, from a legal standpoint, before we could concern ourselves with his advance directive. He explained that he only referred to his advance directive as a tool to help us to understand his current wishes, in view of his difficulties communicating with us.

During the next few days, the family members, the physician, and a few of the staff members who were most closely connected with Mr. White spent a great deal of time with him, trying to understand his wishes. In addition to (repeatedly) asking about the feeding tube, staff tried to ascertain what other treatments he would be willing to receive, depending upon potential future needs. They inquired about antibiotics, cardiopulmonary resuscitation, and a host of other potential treatment options. Mr. White gave inconsistent responses to these questions. When asked if he currently wanted to keep living or preferred to die, he again answered inconsistently. Soon Mr. White was having choking episodes when fed by mouth in addition to rapid weight loss due to inadequate nutritional intake. Without artificial nutrition and hydration through a feeding tube, he would soon die.

Alex impatiently reminded everyone that his father had, when first asked, several times expressed his refusal to receive a feeding tube. However, the physician was ambivalent about whether or not Mr. White was currently capable, so he decided he would meet with him *one last time* to ascertain if he was capable to make a decision to refuse or accept a feeding tube. The rest of the team was worried that if Mr. White was found to be incapable, we would be faced with a dilemma because his two substitute decision-makers disagreed with each other. Brie and Alex were charged with the duty to decide, in accordance with their father's most recently expressed capable wishes, whether or not a feeding tube ought to be inserted.

When Mr. White's physician asked him if he would like to see what a feeding tube looked like, he nodded "yes." After viewing it and having the procedure simply explained, he nodded his head in agreement when asked if he would consent to having one inserted. The physician felt that Mr. White had just expressed a *likely* capable wish. He explained that even though there was some doubt as to his capability to consent, he believed he had a moral and legal duty to err on the side of life. The team agreed. Some said they felt an ethical obligation to try to buy a little more time for Mr. White and his family, especially given his relatively young age. Their hope was that a feeding tube would prolong his life. Everyone was aware that in the best case scenario, he likely had only a few months to live.

Mr. White's son raised the concern that, by extending his life, which possibly the feeding tube would do, his father would likely experience the anguish of suffering through a more progressive stage of his tumor, clearly something he wanted to avoid. After all, he reminded the team that he wrote the advance directive soon after receiving the diagnosis of the tumor, aware of the horrific effects he would experience as the disease progressed. However, the physician reminded him, his father was most likely expressing a capable wish when he agreed to the tube, and therefore he was obliged to follow it. In fact, there is no legal role for the SDM aside from when a patient cannot make a capable decision with respect to this specifically offered treatment. Brie was clearly relieved, while Alex appeared dumbfounded. The feeding tube was inserted.

Mr. White died 5 weeks later, with his twin children at his side. Since the time of his tumor diagnosis, only 3 months had elapsed. His death occurred much earlier than had been predicted.

A number of ethical challenges arose from this case.

Discussion and Analyses

Did Mr. White's Advance Directive Meet The Criteria of Informed Consent?

In the previous chapters, I discussed problems of irreversibility and prediction, as well as related issues of understanding and appreciation, in the context of informed consent. Let us now examine whether the circumstances peculiar to the case of Mr. White offered any particular advantages, as I suspect they might. My rationale follows.

(a) By the time Mr. White met with his lawyer to write his advance directive, he had already received the diagnoses of Alzheimer's dementia and a brain tumor. Likely, his advance directive was better informed, as a result of his understanding and appreciation of the issues he was addressing. It could be argued, however, that this advantage was relevant only to his experience of the early stages of his diseases. New symptoms emerged after the time of constructing his directive and without prior experiential "benefit." Nonetheless, in general, I believe that Mr. White's advance directive was in this sense more informative in comparison to those of others who have at best only their (likely largely ineffective) predictive moral imaginative powers to rely upon.

(b) The time period between the date when Mr. White wrote his advance directive, and the initial circumstance for which it was to be applied, was a mere few days, within which no significant events occurred. Given such a limited time frame, not only was it less likely that his values, interests, and wishes might have changed, it was also less likely that external factors, such as new treatments being made available, would arise.

(c) A sequence of actions occurred that indicated Mr. White understood what an advance directive was supposed to achieve and that he knew which steps to take to enable its process. We know that Mr. White discussed his intention of completing a directive with his nurse ahead of time and agreed to his son initiating the legal consultation. He expressed relief that he would have the chance to express his medical treatment wishes. Since these events occurred while Mr. White was already in care, (unlike in the cases of Mr. Black and Mrs. Black), we had the advantage of being privy to them.

Mr. White's advance directive, however, was not flawless. The concerns listed below would have negatively impacted how informed it was.

(a) Brie was concerned that the lawyer met with her father only briefly (approximately for 20 min), and therefore she surmised he must have rushed him through the process, possibly resulting in his father not having enough time to understand all the issues involved.

I think Brie's concern was a valid one. While it seemed evident that Mr. White understood the main purpose of having an advance directive, it is possible that other pertinent information might not have been conveyed to him. Additionally, he was in the beginning stages of both diseases, and it could be reasonably argued that he really had no appreciation of how he would experience the later stages, particularly if he was to become a happy dementia patient. After all, he wrote his advance directive at a time when he was often angry and frustrated. Had he been informed that a change in his emotions later in time might result in a "happier" experience, it is far from clear that he would have written what he did.[2] On the other hand, given that the co-occurrence of his brain tumor was expected to shorten his life considerably, it would be unlikely that he would experience the more advanced stage of his dementia.

(b) We really did not know how much information Mr. White received about the specifics of his medical diagnoses and management of his symptoms (currently and also with an eye to future months as well). All we knew is that apparently he was told he would likely live for about a year. In this case we were, unfortunately, not able to glean any more information from Mr. White because he was unable to communicate that knowledge to us.[3] It goes without saying that

---

[2] This concern can be generalized to most directives.

[3] In Mr. White's case, there was a lawyer involved in the process, but no permission to contact him was granted. I have subsequently learned that we did retain the legal right to contact him but that likely most lawyers would refuse to reveal that kind of confidential information about their clients.

sharing relevant information with the client is a requisite criterion in order for him to be able to make an informed decision.[4]

(c) Another concern of mine had to do with Mr. White's ability to understand and appreciate all the relevant information, due to impaired cognitive functioning related to his diseases.[5]

Nonetheless, as already mentioned, he certainly demonstrated that he was able to grasp the overall purpose of writing a directive. The fact that he agreed to a meeting with the lawyer alone and was looking forward to it demonstrated some important insight as well. I do not think we have any information that would preclude his understanding and appreciating the information and consequences of his decisions; at least, not to the extent that we could, with confidence, consider his directive to be of no use whatsoever.

Whatever information may have been relayed too scantily, or omitted altogether, we cannot assume he received any less information about the risks and consequences of having an advance directive than would most others. The advantages he had in terms of currently experiencing the medical conditions that most people can only more or less imagine in their minds and the limited time period existing between his having a directive written and its application have already been noted.

To summarize, there are definite strengths to Mr. White's directive. I think that most would agree that prediction, understanding, and appreciation are relevant criteria to consider when assessing the merit of any particular advance directive. We must bear in mind, though, that significant subjective variations will occur when it comes to defining them and in assigning merit, weight, and applicability to any particular case.

Some of the usual concerns were likely pertinent as well, such as whether Mr. White had been given relevant information, including that in the future he might experience dementia very differently than he does now.[6] But we cannot

---

I do not know of any court action that has occurred, but it would be interesting to see what might happen if that approach was explored.

[4] However, there are no such legal requirements when it comes to advance directives.

[5] In Chap. 3, I referred to the belief that many people write advance directives when they are in the beginning stages of their dementia. I identified a potential paradox. Some persons might be perceived to be lacking the requisite capabilities to produce an informed directive; at the same time, being in the early stage presents one with the actual experience of dementia which should result in a heightened level of appreciation and thus make one better informed. Of course, each person's situation is experienced differently and must be understood in its respective context.

[6] This issue may have direct relevance for whether or not Mr. White has the information that *he* requires in order to understand and appreciate the risks and benefits before an informed decision can be made. I already referred to the notion that some dementia patients seem to have happy existences. We do not know if he had been given that information before. We know for a fact that a medical professional did not give him that information at the time his directive was written, though we cannot for certain assume that his lawyer did not impart relevant information, nor can we say with certainty that he did not learn that information from some other source prior to writing the directive. This raises a pertinent question for me: "On what grounds can we say that this particular piece of information has enough relevance to Mr. White's personal situation that it ought to

know if these requirements had been met, let alone be assured that the specific information shared was of the kind that was relevant *for Mr. White*. Without knowing more details regarding both the content and process that Mr. White underwent when he wrote his advance directive, relevant to his values, and without access to objective standards of evaluation (notwithstanding the fact that it is likely not possible to derive objective measures), it is difficult to determine *just how informed* his advance directive was.

I have already recommended that in general we ought to understand the role of the advance directive in situations where the patient is conscious as being corroborative. An advance directive might help us better understand the current experience of the patient to inform treatment decision-making. By usually limiting the conditions of applicability so narrowly and so specifically, hopefully we will have succeeded in reducing the foreseeable risks and negative consequences that might otherwise arise out of its use.

Was Mr. White capable to make an informed decision regarding the feeding tube treatment?

The physician, with the agreement of most of the team, determined he could not reach a conclusion about Mr. White's capacity and decided to keep trying to do so over a number of ensuing days. On the one hand, it may be argued that this question was settled during the very first meeting – that he demonstrated his capacity, and could have been put to rest. On the other hand, in addition to being driven by the best of intentions, the physician's efforts to be thorough through a lengthier process of assessment should be lauded.

Before I identify the reasons why Mr. White was likely capable at the time I referred to above, and before I identify the factors that I believe contributed to the team being uncertain about his capacity status, I will provide a brief review of the legal standard for informed consent in Ontario as well as provide some of my own reflections related to the topic of capacity.

By now we should be clear on what is the legal standard for informed consent to treatment requires, at least in Ontario:

1. Capacity is decision-specific and temporally based. I might not have the capacity that is required to make an informed decision pertaining to brain surgery, but I could perhaps consent to getting my eyes examined. Maybe I cannot make a

---

be considered as pertinent for *him?*" Shouldn't Mr. White be the determiner (at least to some extent) of what kind of information he thinks he needs to be able to make an informed enough decision? His personal values ought to significantly matter here. This issue leads me to the essential topic of what standards are typically used by practitioners when they disclose information to patients, since they are implicated in the process in a very substantial way. While in Ontario no such standard is regulated in the case of advance directives, I have discussed it as it applies to informed consent procedures in the previous case of Mrs. Black.

capable decision about accepting or refusing a particular treatment when I am asked at 9 a.m., but I might be able to do so at 10 a.m. after I have taken my memory medication.

2. The criteria for capacity are supposed to represent objective standards or reference points, but it is up to each respective practitioner to make his own decision, which entails subjective judgments on his part. The concepts "understand" and "appreciate" are themselves vague, often defined differently by practitioners, and influenced by personal and professional biases. In my experience, some practitioners consider both terms to mean the same thing. It is up to the practitioner who is offering the treatment to make the determination about whether or not the patient can satisfy the criteria for informed consent. Two different practitioners at the same time, each understanding capacity to mean something else, could differ in their opinions about the same patient's capacity with regard to the ability to make an informed decision for the same treatment decision. This is not, in my experience, an uncommon phenomenon. And yet the consequences can be profound.

In the previous chapter on the case of Mr. Black, I suggested that the legal criteria for capacity are problematic when it is applied to most people with Alzheimer's dementia beyond the very early stage, because it rules them out of consideration for making choices about their futures or even from having their wishes reflected in what is medically done to them. Furthermore, the criteria do not capture the usual way people with or without dementia make decisions. I prefer a different approach compatible with the following: I might not have full capacity but rather partial abilities in these areas. Other people who know me well can help me to better understand and appreciate what is at stake and/or help me express my values and wishes if I lack the ability to do so. My values ought to guide the decisions that I am helped to make or are expressed for me, if I am unable to do so.

I also stated that only in very rare situations (one example being when a patient with dementia is in an irreversible coma and the advance directive is judged to be the most comprehensive source of information about the patient's values and interests or only source when the patient is relatively unknown) ought an advance directive to be seriously considered. Otherwise, when it happens to largely cohere with the current wishes and values of the patient, it serves to further our understanding of the values and wishes that are presently important to the patient. When we can identify a match between what we believe to be the patient's current wishes and values, with the wishes stated in the advance directive, our confidence tends to be boosted.

In retrospect, I think it is reasonable to believe that Mr. White likely met the standard legal criteria to decide whether or not he wished to receive a feeding tube during the very first meeting it was offered to him. Perhaps it is worth considering that in any event we should not hold Mr. White to the strict application of the legal standard because it does a disservice to the dementia population we serve. Perhaps we ought to have accepted his refusals when first asked, while not being certain about his level of understanding and appreciation; furthermore, he was consistent in his response about endorsing his advance directive wishes as representing his current wishes.[7]

While understanding (from a legal point of view) that his advance directive would have become relevant only if Mr. White was unable to express current capable wishes, some members nonetheless referred to it to emphasize that it was recently written and allied with his current wishes. This alliance, however, requires that Mr. White held the beliefs that acceptance of a feeding tube was incompatible with dying with dignity, and that a feeding tube was a heroic treatment. It is not unreasonable to speculate that Mr. White did hold those beliefs, though we cannot be certain of it. Recall as well, that Alex stated that his father told him many times that he did not wish to continue to live, since the diagnosis of his brain tumor. The combination of these factors I believe should have settled the issue of determining that Mr. White was choosing to refuse receipt of a feeding tube. Yet, I too had some doubts when the issues first surfaced. It is one thing to hear this story and quite another to have been part of its unraveling drama.

When I reflect on why our particular team had trouble accepting Mr. White's initial refusals as capable (let us remember that capacity is the legal standard), and instead opted to continue the process to develop greater clarity, a number of possibilities come to my mind. Before identifying them, I will again recap the salient events that occurred during the initial meeting with the team, Mr. White, and his two children to provide the context.

The first time the physician asked Mr. White if what he wrote in the advance directive reflected what he wanted today, following his recital of it, he responded "yes." Then his two children each asked him the same question, as did two or three staff. He consistently nodded "yes." Each time during this initial meeting that he was offered a feeding tube, he declined. In total, he was asked three or four times, and each time he vehemently shook his head "no." The questions followed a brief but concise description of the risks and benefits. When the physician asked him what he understood about the treatment, he tried to talk but failed. It was difficult to gauge his depth of understanding because of his inability to speak clearly. However, his answers that day were consistent with each other and also as aforementioned, likely cohered with what he had written in his advance directive just a few weeks prior.[8] I therefore anticipated that there would have been agreement that Mr. White likely made a capable decision to reject the feeding tube.

---

[7] It is not unusual practice that consistency of responses (as sole criterion) is considered to be a sufficient (albeit minimal) indicator of capacity in situations requiring decision-making by patients who are marginally or inconsistently capable. Many patients in early stage dementias, and possibly in the moderate phases as well, would likely fit this description. This issue is very worthy of further discussion, I believe, but not one that I can give sufficient attention to in this book.

[8] I have previously suggested that we lower the bar on capacity when it comes to decisions that matter the most. If we had not obtained consistent responses from Mr. White, then I would have relied more on observing his behaviors and actions, trying to glean from them what his values and wishes were. In addition, I think his recently written advance directive would most likely be considered to be good evidence of what his values and wishes were though they should not count as determinative if what he expressed since that time varied significantly. This idea was discussed in the previous case of Mrs. Black.

However, this was not the prevailing view for all at that time. Brie argued with a sense of desperation that her father ought to be given the feeding tube. There was a palpable sense of anxiety on the part of team members who voiced hesitation about what would be the "right thing to do." At the time, I too was somewhat ambivalent about what we ought to do, purely from an ethical perspective, that is, setting aside as much as possible the more prudential worries about managing a dispute between two conjoint SDMs (should their roles of being SDMs be activated if the patient was deemed incapable).

With the brief review of events, as I have reconsidered them, in place, we are now ready to identify and analyze the factors that contributed to what otherwise typically may have been a more straightforward case of a patient refusing treatment. It is only in retrospect that I understand them with more clarity now.[9]

(a) Brie claimed that her father was not psychologically ready to make such a difficult decision due to being traumatized. She wondered if this also affected his capacity to make a decision. She believed that his decision to refuse treatment was consistent with his usual initial reaction of refusing anything "new" and predicted that he would consent to a feeding tube at a later time because he was not yet ready to die.

In my view, Brie's points were certainly not implausible. Plus, she had the advantage of knowing her father much more intimately than did the team.[10] Furthermore, the claim regarding her father's traumatization was truly compelling. After all, Mr. White did receive the devastating news of a second terminal illness, which meant that he likely had only months to live. It is possible that Brie and Alex were also traumatized by the very sad state of affairs and were also not yet emotionally ready for their father to die.

Whenever a family member vehemently protests against a decision, strong emotional reactions, understandably, are aroused on the team. There was no question that staff felt very emotionally pulled by what Brie had stated. Overall, I felt that she had the greatest impact upon the physician who empathically referred to the devastating set of circumstances Mr. White and his children faced. It was obvious the physician was feeling very moved when Brie urged the team to insert a feeding tube with the hopes of buying her father a little more time in order to determine if he would choose otherwise if and when less traumatized.

---

[9] Being unsettled, so to speak, about ethical "determinations" (loosely interpreted) is an occasional experience for me. Not always does clarity come to me during the actual consultation process. Passage of time and reflection may need to occur. However, I still would not call the process "settling" to any great extent.

[10] Mr. White had the somewhat unusual distinction of not having been a long-term patient when all these issues arose. Often I am called to consult on cases where the patients or residents have been living in the respective facility for a number of years and the staff members develop a much more familiar type of relationship with them.

(b) As aforementioned, Alex strongly disagreed with Brie for reasons already cited, even though these may have conflicted with his own emotions or desires. I found his arguments very compelling as well. Brie seemed shaken by their disagreement, having expressed how close she and her brother had always been. Clearly, the staff did not wish to do anything to escalate their conflict and at the same time recognized full well that anything they could have said or done might have unwittingly served to do just that.

(c) The introduction of sibling conflict further raised the level of the team's anxiety. Disagreement between family members is not unusual of course, especially when the stakes are perceived to be so high, and team members can feel ill-equipped to deal with it.[11] We had already witnessed several precedent cases where conflict between family members escalated to the point where relationships were severed, perhaps permanently. Often staff members believe they bear some responsibility for this, and the guilt and distress that result can be quite debilitating. Most unfortunately, the focus on the patient can get derailed by the conflict at hand. Perhaps, saddest of all is that at a time when deep feelings of sadness and loss could be expressed in ways that draw family members closer, including of course quality of time spent with the patient, the opposite is often proven true in situations of high conflict.

Often family conflicts arise in reference to differences about what is perceived to be the most significant or highly held values, interests, or wishes of the patient. I try to normalize this phenomenon. There is much truth in my statement when I tell them, "Even fully (biologically) related siblings never have the same parent." We know how complex and nuanced familial relationships are and how distinctively unique each bond or link is. Considering also how likely it is for different family members to recall past incidents so differently, it is of little surprise that multiple versions of what naively is believed to be the "same and only story" are often generated.

At times I share my own personal story of my family's struggle to determine what treatment my then-critically ill father would have wanted when he was unable to express himself after suffering a stroke. It was very humbling and informative for me to experience the intense moral distress that our patients' families often endure in these kinds of situations, which can easily morph into full-blown crises. Not to be unexpected, my family members also had divergent opinions about the treatment we thought our father would have chosen for himself. I recall how mere *opinions*, initially calmly uttered, quickly transformed into *absolute truths*, loudly asserted, in a matter of seconds when it came to the "evidence" claimed to buttress our individual versions of reality. I remember well the expressions of astonishment on our faces upon hearing from each other what sounded like unfamiliar stories being told by strangers. Of course, when cooler heads prevailed, it becomes quite obvious that the truth of past incidents or character traits was often less important for our joint decision-making than

---

[11] Anger and anxiety levels can easily sky rocket, and complete relationship ruptures between family members have on more than one occasion occurred.

achieving some mutually coherent perception of them. As an ethicist helping family members navigate through their divergent views, I try to use these different perspectives in a positive way. It is an opportunity to begin to talk with the family members about the multiple ways in which the patient can be understood, to open up rather than shut down their conversations. It is important not to alienate any of the family members. While perhaps obvious, it bears repeating that you cannot credibly claim that only one of them is "right" because we are talking about perceptions and beliefs, not absolute truths, about one family member, the patient, according to another. Given how uncertain we can be about our own interests and wishes, it is easy to understand how unreliable anyone else can be about what matters to another. We cannot with confidence say that we are sure about the wishes of the patient, so the best we can do is to try to deliberate a process where as much information as possible can emerge about the values and interests of the patient central to the decision at hand.

(d) This particular team was very committed to trying to reach consensus.[12] While it is the responsibility of the treating practitioner to determine capacity, there is an assumption on this team that "more brains are better than one." This organization rightly believes that decision-making practices are often enriched as a result of input from a diversity of professional values, experiences, and perspectives on the team. It is expected that "everyone shall have a voice," although of course there are mitigating influences such as team power differences that establish the decisional hierarchy, or pecking order so to speak. When all staff members do not agree with the final decision being made (and this is not uncommon across the various healthcare organizations I have worked within), lingering moral distress can result which, if left unresolved, can seriously impact upon the team members' ability to work together and to provide optimal care for their patients. Fortunately, most healthcare facilities that I have been involved with offer the requisite support for comprehensive team deliberations, reflections and debriefing, and subsequent team building to occur.

This particular team in fact did have a significant history of successfully addressing their interdisciplinary team conflicts, which by the way are inevitable. To their credit they had recently participated in a 2-day retreat where external personnel had been hired to work with the group with the goal of enhancing their collaboration skills. Apparently, it had proven to be a positive experience, and the team members were very motivated to continue to strengthen their working relationships. In the case of Mr. White, they were not only trying to meet the best interests of their patient but also respecting their commitment to collaborate as an interdisciplinary team.[13] Much emphasis was put on encouraging each team member to voice his or her opinions on each issue that gets

---

[12] I do not know that it is always best to try to reach a consensus. While this objective may be reached, there may be a cost of members making dramatic compromises of their own personal or professional values. I have witnessed extensive resentment and resulting moral distress that lingered, in some cases, for years. I will say more about this shortly.

[13] These goals are, ideally, mutually compatible and reinforcing.

raised. Where the staff still required support was in feeling comfortable with respectfully challenging each other's ideas. When the doctor first expressed doubt about Mr. White's capacity, I observed through facial and other nonverbal body language that not all agreed. However, no staff member seemed ready to voice a different opinion. While noteworthy, this type of response is not necessarily idiosyncratic to Mr. White's case. The internal dynamics of the interprofessional healthcare team *always* play a role in how decisions are made and what decisions are made, including in relation to patient capacity, and can powerfully impact how differences in opinion are dealt with in regard to the interpretation of an advance directive. This serves to illustrate once again (as was the situation in the previous two cases) the naïveté of supposing that an advance directive in itself has the power to settle, or even strongly constrain, the treatment a patient will receive.

(e) There was difference of opinion among individual team members, and across teams as well, about how much weight ought to be given to a family's interests—or a particular member's interests—when they might conflict with those of the patient.[14,15] Partly this is discipline specific. For example, some healthcare team members due to their specific professional roles are more in contact with families and tend to get to know the family members better than do other team members.[16]

---

[14] Potential conflicts of interests of course also occur between and across multiple stakeholder groups, including and not restricted to family members.

[15] I recall a situation where everybody on the team shared a very different interpretation of an advance directive than did the sole adult child. She held the substitute decision-making authority in this case, as attorney for personal care. The patient had clearly stipulated he would not want any further medical treatment offered or any current ones continued under very specific conditions. He was in an irreversible coma. The staff believed beyond a doubt that the respective conditions were present and that it was time to withdraw his treatments. Nonetheless the daughter refused to give consent to do so, stating that he had since expressed different wishes than what was written in his advance directive to her verbally, prior to going into a coma, and when he was competent, that would be in opposition to not receiving treatment currently or to withdrawing his current treatuments. The team, not knowing the veracity of this, also felt very concerned for the daughter's wellbeing. The daughter was known as someone who lived a marginal existence outside of her deep connection to her only living relative, her father. She herself had had suffered through many losses and traumas in her lifetime. They acknowledged that perhaps she was being truthful. Plus they also knew that her father was likely going to die within a few weeks anyway, and they did not believe that extending his life beyond the time he stipulated in the directive would cause him suffering, given his comatose state. They promised her they would not withdraw any treatments and they would give him any additional ones needed in the future. A couple of the staff members voiced an additional justification. They said they knew their patient to be a gentleman who, above all else, "lived for his daughter." They felt that he would never have wanted a decision to be made that would cause such angst for his daughter. I raise this case in part to demonstrate the complexity and uniqueness of each situation. I also wanted to draw attention to the fact that there are potentially a countless number of factors that influence medical decision-making at any one particular moment in time, and the decisions that involve an advance directive are no exception.

[16] I think it is reasonable to assume that the staff members who best know the family members are also the ones who tend to more often factor the family's best interests into their decision-making, since their interests are better known.

As we have seen, there are many factors that intervene. No two situations are ever alike, and it is often difficult to even identify let alone articulate the multitude of influences that impinge on any decision.

(f) At the time, some members of the team were still ambivalent about whether or not to consider Mr. White to be capable regarding the treatment decision at hand. Alex and Brie's duties as joint substitute decision-makers would not be required unless their father was considered to be incapable to make a specific decision. Only then would their opinions and decisions from a legal standpoint become relevant and applicable. However, there seemed to be a lack of clarity in terms of what roles team members thought Alex and Brie were entitled to assume, partly related to misunderstanding of the role of the substitute decision-maker. It was under these unclear circumstances that lack of consistency occurred, in terms of how team members engaged (or did not) with Brie and Alex and what kind of authority, legal or otherwise, they perceived them to be operating within.

Another factor was also at play. Staff members who perceived Mr. White as capable sought out family members' opinions to help assign meaning to his current wishes and behaviors as well as to ascertain what important values he was currently expressing. We already know, however, that the opinions of family members do not hold any legal clout unless they are officially acting in the capacity of substitute decision-makers (including as attorneys for personal care) and therefore are required to ensure that the directive is complied with. We also know that from a legal point of view that duty was to be assumed by Alex and Brie only when it was believed that Mr. White could not make a current capable decision with respect to the treatment being considered. Nonetheless, some team members interacted with them as family members who know the patient the best. This practice may be commonplace and makes good sense in terms of gaining greater understanding of patients' values, beliefs, and wishes. Other team members who perceived Mr. White to be capable during the initial meeting voiced their strong disapproval of the team's intent in continuing to meet with the children after the patient had left the room, the patient's consent notwithstanding.

The family's views were irrelevant, they reminded us, because the decision was Mr. White's alone, unless he preferred otherwise. Still others who did not perceive him to be capable were interacting with Brie and Alex as his substitute decision- makers and eliciting their assistance with interpreting his advance directive. There were some team members who engaged them as part of the decision-making process, irrespective of their father's level of capacity. The occurrence of inconsistencies, in part maybe due to lack of shared understanding about the legal standards (a problem that can be easily resolved), also portrayed distress about potential gaps that were perceived to exist between selective aspects of the law they were expected to conform with, and what they believed to be good clinical practices. I think this situation highlights the complexities that exist in real-life clinical situations and how challenging and limiting it is to try to apply a legal standard template to them.[17]

(g) This particular physician is a very well-respected and strong member on this team and yields a great deal of influence upon the others. When he expressed doubt about what conclusions to reach about Mr. White's capacity, some others immediately followed suit.

(h) Most staff members seemed to be uncomfortable with Mr. White's decision to refuse treatment. As a consequence, the process was perhaps prolonged.

I noticed a sense of panic in the team that I had rarely before experienced. I recall the meeting we had initially when Mr. White expressed his refusal of the feeding tube. The 30 or 40 min spent together in that meeting room were about the most tense of any consultations I can recall. While typically these sorts of situations can be quite anxiety-laden, this one was different. Over the years, I have seen many patients like Mr. White with mild dementia who make decisions without being able to clearly articulate their understanding of the treatment offered, and/or to not be able to express with absolute certainty an appreciation of it. They may forget what they consented to, they may even forget they consented, but as long as their responses are consistent, their decisions are often accepted as being capable *enough*. Somehow this standard was not extended to Mr. White.[18]

Basically Mr. White made a decision that was uncomfortable to most in the room. Perhaps (and this is solely my own projection and attribution) the discomfort was due mainly because Mr. White was too young, too vulnerable, and too close to the age of many of the staff members.[19] After much reflection, I have come to believe that Mr. White's capacity was likely never really the whole issue (or perhaps it was yet became subverted by our own subjectivity). Yet at the time, none of our decisions seemed fundamentally couched in terms of the factors just discussed. The medical and legal framework of the advance directive, the SDMs, and the assessment of Mr. White's current wishes served as a structure through which our ideas, beliefs, and empathic reactions could be implemented—in a partially acknowledged (and well-intended) form—as it now seems even clearer to me with the benefit of

---

[17] It required quite a bit of time and effort on my part, as well as on the part of the staff, to resolve these inconsistencies. Some of it occurred during the life of the initial consultation; some of it became clarified through debriefing sessions that occurred later; some of it occurred in subsequent consultations with the same team. Notably, differences between team members do not necessarily vanish upon the death of the patient, and processes to continue to attempt to resolve them are an important feature of health team's development.

[18] This "standard" that I refer to may not necessarily uphold the legal criteria for informed consent, strictly speaking. It is at times difficult to determine, given the nuances and somewhat subjective interpretations that necessarily prevail. Nonetheless, it currently is the unofficial default clinical practice standard (more or less) that this particular team has adopted for the population they are working with. Variances likely occur not only between respective teams but between individual healthcare providers as well.

[19] Of course, there are numbers of people who die at a younger age than Mr. White. I imagined that there was a fair amount of subjectivity of values and beliefs being expressed and unintentionally perhaps being projected, especially given that a number of staff were more used to working with a population of patients who were significantly older than Mr. White.

time and reflection. Additionally, given the mixed motivations earlier mentioned, it is possible that the physician was simply conflicted (understandably) and hoped for *something* decisive to happen through the creation of a prolonged evidential situation through repeated asking. He may have also been hoping to justify a team-coherence choice, especially in the face of what was appearing to be an unpopular/distressing patient-autonomy choice.[20][21]

A question I am left with is how we, as a team, can become more aware of our own projections, needs, beliefs, and biases at the time so that we can be better in control of them. Often, after a consultation, we will allow some time to pass and then we will meet again to share reflections about how the process of ethical decision-making occurred, critiquing how legal, moral and professional standards and guidelines were met, how to better support each other, etc. These types of sessions often stimulate heightened self-awareness and stronger team relationships. We engage in deeper discussions about our decision-making processes and challenge our own and each other's ideas about how we might approach a similar situation (such as Mr. White's) in a different and perhaps more morally reasoned fashion. As an ethicist, I often play an integral role in the facilitation of these sorts of reflections. While these sorts of experiences provide useful lessons, retrospectively, it remains challenging to know how to gain insight into problematic ethical proceedings as they are currently unfolding. In retrospect I realized that I may very well have benefitted from some assistance from colleagues at that time who were external to this particular situation and likely in the position to render more objective perspectives. I, the ethicist, am not immune from projection of my own preferences, values, and biases.

Additional Ethical Issues

We have already discussed the issue about the status of Mr. White's capacity when he was initially questioned about his wishes regarding a feeding tube and questioned if he likely should have been deemed capable and his refusal ought to have been honored. Had these conclusions been reached by all of us back then, it is fair to assume that there would have been no reason to probe further. But we also know that the physician was ambivalent about whether or not Mr. White was capable and

---

[20] I thank Professor Tim Kenyon, Brock University, Canada, for his insights about potential motivators.

[21] It strikes me as well that some of the dynamics being played out by the family members were isomorphic to those of the team. Disagreements about some of the same issues (capacity status, relevance of use of advance directive) reverberated between staff members and between family members also. Evidence of this sort of parallel processes occurring is certainly not exclusive to this particular case. Often when I observe this phenomenon, I identify it to the team members, the aim being to facilitate greater self-understanding of their own emotions, values, and biases, in the hopes of not projecting them onto the respective case, as well as enhanced insight into their team dynamics.

that the daughter and some team members did not deem Mr. White to unequivocably be capable.

Let us take the stance that the facts of this case were such that it was indeed very difficult to determine Mr. White's capacity status when presented with the treatment option. The reality of his children holding opposing views, however, remains a constant.

Given this scenario, would the physician's pursuant actions have been morally justifiable?

To answer this question, I will first present a narrative review of the series of events that unfolded at the time.

Over the ensuing days, Mr. White quickly regressed both from a physical and a cognitive point of view. The physician, with the assistance of other staff and Brie and Alex, continued to ask Mr. White if he wished to receive a feeding tube. At this point in time, unlike earlier, he responded inconsistently, meaning that occasions where he nodded in agreement to accept the feeding tube were often trailed and, mere seconds later, by shaking his head in disagreement.[22] It was becoming increasingly difficult for me to discern the basis upon which the physician and other staff would be prepared to make a settled determination about Mr. White's capacity and finally cease repeatedly asking him the same questions. If indeed acceptance of the tube was the only response the team was prepared to accept, I had trouble understanding why none of his affirmative responses were acted upon. Perhaps the team was hoping that Mr. White would express his acceptance of the tube at least twice consecutively. However, doing so would certainly be inconsistent with how they responded earlier when Mr. White did express consistent responses across a number of occasions (when he repeatedly shook his head "no"). As mentioned earlier, in clinical practice, it is not unusual for me to observe that consistency of responses (even in the absence of clear and consistent evidence of understanding and appreciation) is deemed to be sufficient to accord the patient with "sufficiently enough" capacity. However, lack of such consistency did not result in decreeing Mr. White to be incapable.

At the time, I also anticipated that one of two reactions would likely be forthcoming from the physician. While both options shared the same belief, that being currently Mr. White could not make a capable decision, the first one entailed the doctor referring back to the first meeting when his patient consistently expressed refusal of the tube. In light of how much Mr. White had cognitively regressed since then, I imagined he would decide retrospectively that his previous expressions were in fact

---

[22] Perhaps not surprisingly, team members assigned different meanings to his inconsistency. Some felt that it was a normal ambivalence. Others felt that we were responsible for his alleged "incapacity" that was "induced by the discomfort" of repeatedly questioning him about his wishes. Others were more inclined to blame his dementia for his inconsistent responses.

capable ones and that as a result no feeding tube ought to be inserted. A palliative care plan of treatment would be put in place. The second option was that the physician would evoke the law requiring that we defer to Alex and Brie as the joint powers of attorney to ensure compliance with the advance directive, given that capable current wishes could not be obtained. This option would prove challenging if they continued to disagree about the applicability of the directive to the circumstances at hand.[23] Adhering to the wishes of the advance directive would likely also have resulted in Mr. White dying sooner than later, a state of affairs perhaps undesirable to some.

To my surprise at the time, though, neither approach was taken. The physician spent a couple more days speaking to Mr. White's children, eliciting stories about him from the past, in order to develop an appreciation of the kinds of values, beliefs, and interests that seemed important to him. Soon after, he thought that if he showed Mr. White what a feeding tube looked like and tried to indicate how it would be inserted, perhaps then the patient would be able to make a decision.[24] So, that is in fact what he did. Mr. White looked at the physician, smiled at him, and nodded in agreement. "Great!" the physician enthusiastically responded and noted that he felt this was an indication of an "informed enough" consent. A feeding tube was inserted.

---

[23] To briefly review, Brie had argued that her father could not have made an informed decision when the directive was written, because likely he was rushed through the process without enough information to consider and was also depressed at the time. If Brie was to continue to argue in this vein, then in effect she would be discrediting the use of the directive altogether. Alex, on the other hand, believed his father was capable when he wrote the directive and that clearly his specific words unquestionably meant he would not agree to a feeding tube. He also thought his expressions at the first meeting were capable when he refused the feeding tube. While there is no legal reason to demonstrate coherence between his capable wishes at the first meeting and what he wrote in the directive, the symmetry here was not lost on him. I think most people do view repetition of wishes as some sort of indication that these wishes are important to the person expressing them and ought to be honored. It could be perceived as a compelling argument to make.

[24] It was unclear to me if the physician assumed that by showing the patient the medical equipment, he would be better able to grasp the concepts involved and thus aid his cognition and/or if the physician presumed he had the requisite cognitive abilities but needed to be better informed, that is, the patient just needed more information. Either way, I think what the physician was doing was trying to assist Mr. White to make a more informed decision. Provision of this kind of help reinforces the importance of valuing patients' rights to make decisions that matter for them. It speaks to the attempt to avoid the binary approach where you are either capable or you are not. Capacity is located on a continuum, and it is not a static concept. Of interest, British Columbia (Canada) has passed a law a few years ago that obliges healthcare providers to "communicate with the adult in a manner appropriate to the adult's skills and abilities", and "may allow the adult's spouse, or any relatives or friends, who accompany the adult and offer their assistance, to help the adult to understand or to demonstrate an understanding of the matters…". *Health Care (Consent) and Care Facility (Admission) Act* [R.S.B.C. 1996] c. 181. There is a commitment to assisting persons with their capacity that seems to cohere to the notion of relational autonomy, as I discussed earlier. I look forward to learning how this law translates into everyday clinical practice. For further readings in assisting others with capacity, see Lazare, Benaroyo, and Guy Widdershoven, "Competence in Mental Health Care: a Hermeneutic Perspective," *Health Care Analysis* 12, no. 4 (Dec 2004): 297.

When I spoke with the physician afterward, he indicated that to feel comfortable with a decision either way, he needed to know more about Mr. White. When queried about why he had not originally accepted Mr. White's consistent responses to refuse a feeding tube, he said that he was worried about his patient's ability to *really* appreciate the consequences given how traumatized he was and that he also felt that the decision ought to be understood in a larger context. He therefore sought more personal information from the family members. He also remarked that usually he gets to know his patients over a longer period of time and was feeling disadvantaged to help him. His goal was to "buy more time" in order to learn more about him. In addition, he was hoping that Alex and Brie might bridge their disagreement gap and be able to share more of their insights about their father in a calmer, reflective, non-combative way. Again, we note the role that others' preferences and ideas play relative to the implementation and interpretation of the advance directive. The physician in question in this situation was undoubtedly well-meaning, and I came to believe, very thoughtful and deliberative in his approach. At the same time, not being an expert in the legal or philosophical ramifications of advance directive writing for the question of patient autonomy, he held the position of gatekeeper for the dispensation of patient autonomy on his particular healthcare team.

I think it is also important to consider the question of whether the moral comfort of staff ought to be somehow factored into decision-making processes. The short answer is "yes." How that ought to happen and to what extent, in the face of other interests (including of course those of the patient, the family members, other patients, etc.), require a depth of discussion and analysis that is beyond the scope of this book. Nonetheless, I will share a few brief thoughts.

I think that we often become consumed with the ethical duties and responsibilities owed to patients without paying enough attention to those owed to the practitioners. When we analyze case scenarios, it is important to not exclude practitioners' experiences from our moral lens. As an ethicist, I feel an obligation to try to understand what values are driving their opinions and decisions. The attending physician in the case of Mr. White believed that the law ought to be considered a minimal, not optimal standard when it comes to professional codes of conduct and application of medical standards. Like most professionals I encounter, he felt a heightened moral duty to deliver care in a way that was sensitive to the particularities of each individual patient, in accordance with their own personal values. He was not satisfied with trying to apply only the legal standard of capacity in this case.[25] It did not seem quite right to him. While the approach he assumed seemed rather arbitrary to me, at least initially, he reported to me that there was an intuitive sense of purpose and direction to what he did. By interviewing Mr. White's children on several occasions, he was trying to put together a picture of his patient that was larger than the immediate snapshot he took at the first meeting. He wanted to learn more about Mr. White's values and how they might be applied to the current situation, partly through the

---

[25] He certainly was not trying to violate the legal standard. It seemed to me that he was trying to negotiate meeting at least the minimum standard of the law, coupled with his own ethical standard.

children's eyes and through observing Mr. White's behavior over a number of days. He was struggling to understand how the particular decision about accepting or refusing a feeding tube would cohere (or not) with what Mr. White valued at the time, how it could be seen as "his" decision, and how he could be as sure as possible that Mr. White's choices were being honored. The doctor wanted to understand Mr. White's decision(s) in light of his relationships with his children, in accordance with how he was experiencing his brain tumor and dementia, and in respect to any desires that could be gleaned about how he wanted to live his life and the kind of death he wanted to have.

This physician needed to conduct the rather protracted process he undertook, in order for him to feel he was acting in accordance with *his* sense of professionalism. And he required support to do so. Fortunately for him, he was accorded a great deal of influence and power by his team. He was highly respected and had developed a great deal of trust with his colleagues. They felt comfortable (enough) with going along with what he was doing, even though they were not always able to understand and/or necessarily be in agreement with him. As one of his team members commented, "I trust his process." However, there are always other team members who feel that their particular professional approaches and related values and beliefs are not being honored to the same extent as those of others. It becomes quite an interdisciplinary challenge for me to encourage each team member's individual voices to be respected and, at the same time, to find a way to collectively reach a justifiable ethical decision. It is important that staff interests and perspectives are acknowledged and seriously considered and that they believe this to be the case. Otherwise, organizational policies and approaches will not be sustainable. At the end of the day, organizations want to put into place structures that support staff engagement with patients with little risk of quick burnout, often due to moral distress created by staff feeling impotent to contribute to patient welfare. If staff believes that their input are of little concern, there may be a tendency to emotionally withdraw themselves from their patients, which may result in less than optimal patient care experiences.

Now I am ready to address our question pertaining to the ethical nature of the process the physician undertook (with the alteration being that Mr. White's capacity when assessed initially was difficult to determine).

(a) Even if we accept that it was reasonable to be ambivalent about Mr. White's capacity, should the physician have continued to repeatedly ask him the same questions about his wishes and to apply his own interpretative methodology to his responses? It appeared to be obvious that for the physician at no given time, except for the very last one when he elicited an affirmative response from Mr. White, could this issue be settled, regardless of how he answered. Initially, there seemed to be no particular legal or professional standard or rationale that could ground the reason why the physician chose the particular occasion he did to accord Mr. White with capacity. Sometimes, going on a fact-finding mission, so to speak, serves the purpose of clarifying or settling an issue. But in this case, the reverse also could have seemed to be true. What it perhaps ought to have clarified is that Mr. White was becoming increasingly ambivalent and/or incapable. The protracted series of questioning allowed for more opportunities to witness Mr. White's inconsistent responses. The question becomes what ought the team and SDMs do in the face of such current inconsistency? In this particular situation, we had pretty compelling evidence of the patient's very recent wishes to abstain from intervention that was life prolonging and to mitigate his pain as much as possible. I think the argument that his advance directive ought to have been complied with was not an unreasonable one.

(b) It is important to bear in mind that this particular physician is often rightfully lauded for the respect and dignity he treats his patients with and for how he committed he is to honoring the values and beliefs they hold. In fact the qualities inherent in the kind of process he undertook here (including being thorough, engaging the patient and significant others in ways that illuminate the patient's values and beliefs, consideration of the patient's interests that reach beyond medical interests) are usually evident in most of his interactions with his patients. However (and remember that in this version we are imagining that Mr. White did not at any time after he wrote his advance directive express consistency of wishes) as mentioned above, it is fair to question if Mr. White's affirmative nodding of his head when he was shown the feeding tube should have been accorded any exalted meaning over and beyond that given to any of his previous and inconsistent responses. In part, due to the physician's trustworthy reputation, his approach and conclusions were not challenged by others, and that may have been proved to be somewhat unhelpful, though certainly well intended.

We have already established that most advance directives create more problems than they solve but that in the case of Mr. White, his advance directive was somewhat exceptional in a couple of important and positive ways. We know that it was written very recently and at a time when Mr. White was already in the throes of his diseases, though seemingly early enough to still retain most of his cognitive faculties. Given the combination of the inconsistencies he expressed when questioned by his physician, along with the moral ambiguity on the part of the team and the dissension between the SDMs, I think it would have been reasonable to strongly consider his advance directive, especially given its enhanced status, relative to most other directives the team would have encountered in the past.

I think it is fair to ask if we honored Mr. White's interests and values when we kept asking him the same question even though he stated on several occasions that he did not want a feeding tube. Subsequently he became more impaired and could not consistently express his wishes. It is difficult to absolutely endorse the appropriateness of inserting a feeding tube at that time when he had previously stated he did not wish one and never demonstrated any change of heart or gave us justification that would have compelled us to overrule his initial wishes. I cannot however stress enough that this case was extremely challenging on a number of fronts, and many dynamics were at play. The care team's actions and decisions in *retrospect* are being reviewed with the luxury of time and greater objective reality. The intent is not to challenge them in a critical fashion—they are in fact to be lauded on many fronts—but to emphasize the complexity and subjectivity that existed, as expected, and commonly experienced throughout healthcare organizations. The end goal is to be able to become more in tune with our own values, beliefs, and biases and their impact upon our decision-making. Only with greater self-awareness can our own projections be made transparent to ourselves, releasing us (even partially) from their hold.

(c) When Brie called after her father died, she felt that the three of them were well served by his receipt of the feeding tube because it allowed them more time together before he died. However, we could not have known earlier that this outcome was going to occur and necessarily imply that we "did the right thing" according to Mr. White. The feedback from Brie served to reinforce a perception at the time that in fact we did do the "right thing." Any positive future outcomes that may have occurred should not necessarily be mistaken as evidence of that.

What would have happened if Mr. White's current wishes were considered incapable?

From a legal point of view, the SDMs—Alex and Brie—were required to ensure that their father's advance directive was being followed.

Mr. White used terms such as "dying with dignity" and "no heroic measures" which are vague and open to different interpretations. He did not elaborate on the values or beliefs underlying these statements. He did not discuss his advance directive with anyone afterward, as far as we know, and the process he engaged in with the attorney was brief. There was a concern about why Mr. White did not reference his current diseases, although others felt that was a fairly standard omission. It is also true that Mr. White seemed to be in a panic when he wrote it and may also have not been capable to write it. Did he understand and appreciate the consequences of writing this advance directive? How informed was he and could he truly have consented to its application?

We already know that Brie did not consider this directive to be credible because Mr. White was likely incapable (for emotional reasons, and possible cognitive decline) when he filled it out and he did so in a seemingly rushed, impulsive way. We also knew that Alex felt that the advance directive was applicable, borne of genuine wishes and consistent with what his father had been saying to him over a period of months. And let us remember that Mr. White did go to the bother of writing it and had done so very recently.

While the terms "dying with dignity" and "no heroics" are quite vague and general, nonetheless the overall tone of the advance directive was to prevent intrusive interventions. It did not agree to interventions, other than pain control, although in general it was lacking in specificity. I tended to agree with Alex who insisted that the pervading theme was "do less, not more."

Is a feeding tube a heroic measure and/or an intervention that defies a death with dignity?

Most team members believed that in their interpretation, the use of a feeding tube in this situation would not be inconsistent with a dignified death, mainly because they understood that to keep the patient alive, he would require nutrition and hydration, and to offer these to him orally would result in him choking. Either he would choke to death (not viewed by them as a death with dignity) or he would require medical intervention that would be likely irreversible, largely immobilizing, and apt to result in him being even more physically compromised. In their opinion, this would not be acceptable, as he did not say he wanted everything done to preserve his life. It is interesting that the team did not view the feeding tube to be an undignified death, as usually they are concerned with prolonging suffering, and rarely is a tube considered to be an appropriate comfort measure. This is part of the aggregate argument that there were other values and beliefs at play in the assessment of Mr. White's case. As well, some noted that because Mr. White's physical limitations denied him the usual means of eating and drinking, artificial hydration and nutrition should be considered bare necessities, not as medical treatment interventions. This interpretation however flies in the face of usual medical practice guidelines that define artificial hydration and nutrition as medical treatment. A further layer to the complexity is brought by the cultural/social/relational meanings of receiving food, being fed, and eating with others. One of these meanings, which we the team neglected to discuss, was the symbolic meaning of food for Mr. White, given his long-established career as a chef. Specifically, what would it mean to him to no longer savor the taste of food in his mouth, given his personal sense of identity as a chef?

Nonetheless, Alex disagreed with the team's interpretation that insertion of a feeding tube was consistent with a "death of dignity" for his father. He felt that application of the feeding tube was inconsistent with Mr. White's own fairly clearly expressed wish to die with dignity—in whatever sense *he* meant. I also think that if we think of heroic measures as those taken despite very grave consequences to other aspects of one's health or quality of life, then the feeding tube likely qualifies as heroic.

The point I am trying to reemphasize here is that there are an indeterminate number of equally plausible interpretations that could be legitimately claimed. In addition, different contexts or circumstances may be cited to justify respective claims. Brie's insistence that her father receive the tube seemed to be independent of any concern that it cohere with his wishes in the advance directive, either because she did not believe that the directive ought to be considered as relevant in the first place for reasons aforementioned or possibly because a higher interest was driving her insistence.[26]

---

[26] The nub of Brie's insistence seemed to be to keep her father alive for as long as possible because he was "not yet ready to die".

It is worth noting how challenging most ethical decision-making is when it involves the topic of eating and drinking. There are a few reasons for this. One is the uncertainty (briefly mentioned above) about whether eating and drinking are actually medical interventions or necessities of life. If the latter, then it is not open for negotiation, and nutrition must be offered. Everyone *must* be fed. In many of the organizations I have worked with, there is some sort of policy that stipulates that food and drink that are given through artificial means (such as with a feeding tube) constitute a medical intervention. However, even setting aside the problems that any trained philosopher could raise for this definition (Is a fork an artificial means of delivery? How could pureeing food be more artificial than braising it in a tomato sauce?), this concept often flies in the face of the moral comfort zone of many families, patients, and staff members. There are huge cultural, emotional, and social factors at play when we think about our loved ones in relationship to eating and drinking. Helping an infant or toddler to eat is one of the most widely shared and emotionally bonding associations that humans have with dependency and familial attachment. Withholding such assistance for a dependant is a horrible choice, fraught with emotional significance. Many times, family members toss around the term "starving my loved one to death" when they hear about removal of feeding tubes or a plan to stop trying to get the patient to eat when he or she refuses. Visceral reactions of this sort are prevalent whenever issues related to nutrition and hydration are involved. Often family members, personal support workers, or close friends are the ones to assist with feeding. There is no doubt that the act of providing sustenance for life to a loved one is an emotional ritual of bonding that they are often loathe to relinquish.

Undoubtedly the factors influencing medical treatment decisions related to nutrition and hydration are complex and nuanced. It is important that they be identified so that the appropriate structures of support can be provided. Nonetheless, as compelling as any of them might have been in this particular case, I think it would have been wrong to have allowed them priority if we believed that Mr. White's directly expressed wishes to the team to not receive a feeding tube, and/or if his advance directive wish was meant to be understood that according to him, a feeding tube would be a heroic act and therefore a treatment he would not want. Throughout the many years, I have worked as an ethicist, in a number of different healthcare organizations, I have witnessed several other similar situations where a feeding tube has been inserted, when it was questionable if doing so was against the wishes of the patient as stated in an advance directive. In all these cases, complexity of issues existed, with the additional layer of challenges related to nutrition and hydration.[27]

---

[27] I refer to another past case. An elderly patient with mild cognitive impairment had previously written an advance directive while capable, stipulating that, in the event she were to become incapable and had a condition that was incurable and terminal, she denies any medical intervention including but not limited to feeding tubes, antibiotics, cardiopulmonary resuscitation, ventilation, and surgery. The time comes when she has trouble swallowing, she is too weak to express her wishes, and her nutrition intake is very low. The daughter is demanding that a feeding tube be inserted if medically indicated. Insertion of a feeding tube is medically indicated in this case to avoid imminent death. However, the patient's advance directive specifies refusal of this treatment,

Did the SDM contribute value to the advance directive in this case? Does it more generally?

As in each of the other chapters, the issue of the role of the SDM is also central to an analysis of Mr. White's case. This enables me to draw together some more general and cumulative thoughts on the functions and pitfalls of the SDM in our current system.

Let us recall that in the province of Ontario a person's wishes are not interpreted by the physician or other practitioners as may be the case elsewhere in other jurisdictions. It is the legal obligation of the SDM to do so. Recall also that in Ontario the advance directive is not legally viewed as a document of informed consent to treatment. Rather, it is a document of expressed wishes. It is up to the SDM to determine if the wishes are applicable to the current situation. If so, then the duty of the SDM is to ensure that the directive wishes are complied with. It is the SDM who gives or refuses to give informed consent accordingly. On the basis of the cases we've examined, some likely problems with this conception of the SDM's role may be identified.

(a) The SDM may not understand the role. I have encountered a significant number who think their role is simply to decide for the patient, not on the patient's behalf. In their defense, the distinction can be subtle; some substantial explanation and training may be needed to clarify it.

(b) Often, the SDM is unable to understand the wishes expressed and/or has difficulties with their interpretation. We have already discussed the problems of wishes being too vague, too general, or too specific. We already know that there can be a significant amount of subjective interpretation required. It goes without saying that unless there is substantial understanding of the wishes, it is not possible to be able to determine *if they are applicable to the current situation* (notwithstanding that the meaning of this clause is unclear).

(c) Different SDMs apply different interpretations to the phrase "applicable to the current situation."[28]

---

according to the majority of the team. The daughter is the attorney for personal care. The physician senses that the daughter is very anxious and distressed about the likelihood of her mother's imminent death (the mother does not have sufficient nutrition to live more than a couple of weeks). The physician agrees to put in a feeding tube. The attending nurse was the one to most assertively challenge the decision. "After all," the nurse stated, "the situation the patient had described in the directive is the one she is currently in, so there is no question it must be followed." The physician argued that the patient was not necessarily in the terminal (end) stage of her disease and thus the directive was not applicable now. However the nurse countered that the directive was referring to a terminal disease, not a terminal stage of a disease. The doctor argued that the patient had written the word "condition" not "disease," which in her opinion more rightly aligns with the idea of "stage," while the nurse vehemently disagreed and argued that the word "condition" has much more to do with the idea of "disease" than it has to do with the idea of "stage" and so on and so forth. Additionally, there was no definitive diagnosis attributed to her cognitive decline. The physician reminded the nurse and the rest of the team that the interpretation and application of the advance directive was the obligation of the daughter who shared his interpretation.

[28] I have been unable to find any interpretation of this clause. A lawyer I consulted in Ontario who would likely be versed on this advised me that no such legal definition exists in Ontario.

I suggest that if the current situation is *appreciably* changed from the initial situation which existed at the time of writing the directive, then in all likelihood the wish is no longer applicable.[29] We face the question of determining what "*appreciably* changed" means. It is no surprise that this term is subject to a wide range of interpretations. My own work experience confirms this, as do examples we have examined already.

The case of Mrs. Black is a good example—better, perhaps, than the case of Mr. White.[30] Mrs. Black wanted to receive no medications other than for pain control when she could no longer recognize her family members as a result of an irreversible disease. Her wish should not be applied to circumstances that are appreciably changed (or different) than those she had specified as being relevant.[31] For example, it would be obviously wrong to offer only comfort medications while she still recognizes her family. The circumstance of being able to recognize them is obviously different than the circumstance of not being able to recognize them, although in clinical reality recognition speaks to degrees and fluctuations.[32]

I also suggest it is reasonable to claim that the "disappearance" of a previous circumstance is an appreciable change. For example, let us imagine that after she wrote her directive, all of Mrs. Black's relatives were killed in a car accident, and therefore they no longer existed. One of the requisite conditions to which the wish ought to have been applied has vanished, so to speak. It is obvious that family members would have to be in existence as a prior condition to being recognizable as family members.[33] The absence of this condition would render the previous capable wish inapplicable.

---

[29] My starting position is that situations practically *have* to change in *some* way over time. Also see Ralf Jox, "Revocation of Advance Directives," In Advance Directives, ed. Peter Lack, Nikola Biller-Andorno and Susanne Brauer (New York: Springer, 2014), 81. "A person writing an advance directive makes certain assumptions not only about future states of health and the effects of medical treatment, but also about her future mental state, well-being, needs and wishes. If these assumptions turn out to have been false, an important pillar supporting the anticipatory treatment preferences crumbles, rendering the advance directive inapplicable to the current situation...this judgment of applicability is probably the most intricate challenge of dealing with anticipatory statements—all the more so if the patient cannot communicate verbally but only exhibits some kind of behavior that may be interpreted as reflecting the patient's wishes."

[30] Mr. White's advance directive assumes that he is currently in the circumstances he wishes to have his wishes applied to, so appreciable changes in his circumstances were not one of the ethical challenges we confronted.

[31] I use the words "circumstance" and "situation" interchangeably.

[32] Criteria that people use to define recognition vary as well. It is understandably often very distressing for family members and friends to acknowledge and accept that they may not be recognized by the patient. It is not unusual for the family members to claim that the patient does recognize them, in deference to what the staff believes. This issue is exacerbated if recognition of family members is a condition for which an advance directive wish is to be applied, such as in the case of Mrs. Black.

[33] There are, of course, other ways for the family members to be recognized, such as by viewing of their photos.

What should be the determination, however, if the same family in question miraculously survived the car crash but the cure for dementia was believed to be "on the horizon"? Should her previous capable wish be applicable to this situation? According to the criteria that I have suggested, I think we would have a compelling claim of inapplicability to this hypothetical scenario as well. The existence of this new fact of reality renders the current situation dramatically different from the previous one, when the respective wish was expressed.

Mrs. Black became a happy person with dementia. Let us imagine that dementia remained incurable and that at the time she wrote her directive, she believed that dementia could cause only misery. She did not receive information to the contrary that could have been made available to her and that may have resulted in her not expressing the same wish. Should the present situation of being "happy" be considered to be an appreciable change from the circumstances of which she wrote in her directive? This particular scenario addresses the prediction problem that is raised throughout this book. It is no surprise that I would argue that this is exactly the kind of circumstance where the applicability clause has its most relevance. However and not surprisingly, I received opposing answers when I asked lawyers whether a conclusion of inapplicability in this case would be justified. There are no formalized standards, and this is a mixed blessing. On the positive side, it allows for each case to be addressed within its own unique context. However, of concern is that there is no formal accountability framework to which SDMs are held.[34]

Interpretation variation and inconsistency issues aside, the requirement of SDMs to consider this applicability clause has powerful effects. If the reversal of a wish is interpreted as releasing patients from their self-imposed and possibly Procrustean constraints, then this would seem to be a good thing. Theoretically, this could be the panacea we were all waiting for! However, as explained earlier, we cannot know how each patient would experience this effect. Nor can patients know this in advance. The situation becomes even more complex when we factor in not just what the patients said they wished but how they each wanted or expected their advance directive to be applied. Rarely do we know individual patient's preferences in this regard. This complication is addressed in an upcoming paragraph.

Regardless, SDMs are faced with wishes that have to be deemed as either being applicable or not. Certainly some patients would not have wished for what they did if they had been able to accurately predict the future (which of course nobody could do). In my experience, if SDMs are uncomfortable with consenting to the wishes (in the context of denial of treatment), claim may be made that the wishes are not applicable to the current situations. Of course there are a vari-

---

[34] A debate about the mixed blessing could go something like this. One person (rightly) argues that having a standard will not get rid of the subjectivity of interpretation that will occur when trying to apply it to a specific case. And that same person may or may not agree that "wiggle room" is a good thing. Another might claim that, notwithstanding the claim that subjectivity of interpretation cannot be entirely eliminated, at least a standard would set some guidance and direction to SDMS.

ety of reasons why any SDMs might refuse to give consent. In my clinical opinion, the two most common ones are that they are not emotionally ready to lose the patients[35] and that the giving of consent is contrary to the best interests of the patients *now*. Given that many SDMs tend to have close emotional ties with the patients, often these two reasons coexist. This combination tends to result in powerful assertions being expressed. Given that most people in healthcare are aware of the prediction concerns inherent in directives and that a predisposed default to life bias generally exists, SDMs usually do not necessarily face many obstacles if they refuse to consent to the wishes (of not receiving life-prolonging or life-sustaining treatment). When you factor in the lack of clarity about what "applicability to the current situation" means, it is not difficult to imagine that even the thinnest or vaguest reason for overruling the wishes might qualify as justification. In such circumstances, the "wiggle room" might allow for a quick annihilation of the wish by the SDMs. The "wiggle room" that this clause (of applicability) allows is the potential antidote to the directive itself.

Earlier I referred to further complications surrounding the lack of knowledge about how patients intended their directives to be used. I raise this because intentions should be considered to be part of the circumstances from within which the directives were produced. The relevance of the patient's intentions (unfortunately, often unknown) to the process of substitute decision-making is about to become clear.[36]

Let us imagine that a particular SDM decides that a patient's wish is, in fact, not applicable. Let us again consider the case of Mrs. Black but in the following altered context. Her SDM, the son, has been convinced by the team that his mother's wish does not apply to the current situation, because she did not have the benefit of knowing she might possibly become happy despite or perhaps due to her dementia. The son feels torn, however, because after all, his mother did express that wish. And he struggles with feelings of guilt because he has disappointed her by not complying with it. After all, it is reasonable to assume she had expected her wish to be complied with. But (and this came as surprising news to me when I first learned about it) often, this is *not necessarily* the case. Apparently, we should *not* presume that the author of the directive necessarily expects or even wants the directive to be followed. Research indicates a wide range of variability in terms of how flexible an approach a patient wishes or expects their SDMs to assume. Some want or expect that their directives will be strictly adhered to. On the other hand, others prefer that they be considered as informative, but not determinant.

---

[35] Rarely in my experience do SDMs acknowledge their emotional lack of readiness aloud. Many also struggle very much with the emotional loss they are feeling, but do not necessarily act these feelings out in terms of the decisions they are making. See Robert Olick, "On the Scope and Limits of Advance Directives and Prospective Autonomy," Advance Directives, ed. Peter Lack, Nikola Biller-Andorno and Susanne Brauer (New York: Springer, 2014) 66. He states that SDMs may not honor the patient's wishes because of "an inability to let go."

[36] The relevance of *not* knowing the patient's intent will also become clear.

(d) On a related note, many patients want their SDMs to not feel slavishly bound to follow the wishes they have expressed in their directives but rather prefer that they use their own discretion in how final decisions will be made.[37] Of this group, some specify that they want decisions to be made only according to their present interests.[38] It is not always clear how broad a range of interests the authors intended the SDMs to consider. Some patients want only their medical interests to be what drives the decisions being made on their behalf, while others expect that other interests related to their values and beliefs be considered as well.

Allowing for flexibility of approaches seems like a reasonable idea. However, one problem is that often the SDMs are not informed about how the patients expected or wanted their directives to be used.[39] One way to help remediate the problem would be for the patients to address their preferences of approaches within the advance care directive document itself. Directives generally concentrate on *what* their wishes are and *when* they wish them to be applied but are relatively scant on *how* they would like the decisions to be made. Nonetheless, even if they were documented, we still could not predict that these wishes or expectations have remained stable over time. I assume they are subject to the same kind of potential variability as are treatment wishes.

So, when we think about the altered case where Mrs. Black's son decided in accordance with the views of the team, and not in compliance with his mother's directive wishes per se, all his angst may have been for naught. Ultimately, if his mother happened to be one of the patients who wanted or expected that her SDM would not necessarily follow the treatment wishes, then, paradoxically, he may very well have done just what she had wanted!

In the modified scenario, when Mrs. Black's son did not agree to follow her wish to *not* receive treatment, at least two kinds of reasons could have been given. The first was that the previous wish did not apply to the current situation. This reason is directly related to the prediction problem. If it does not make sense to apply a wish from the past because of lack of applicability, there is the option of searching within Mrs. Black's directive for another wish that might

---

[37] In a recent paragraph, I had depicted the SDMs to be in a potentially heroic role where they could unbind the patients from their slavish wishes; now we are learning that authors of directives have a desire to release their SDMs from feeling slavishly bound to carry out the wishes they (the authors) have enslaved themselves to. Ultimately, it appears that the advance directive authors are trying to have their own shackles removed, via the assistance of their SDMs. For more details about patients' expectations of their SDMs in the context of deviating from their wishes, see Jeffrey T. Berger, Evan G. DeRenzo, and Jack Schwartz, "Surrogate Decision Making: Reconciling Ethical Theory and Clinical Practice," *Annals of Internal Medicine,* no. 149 (2008): 48–53; L.K. Fellows, "Competency and Consent in Dementia," *Journal of the American Geriatrics Society* 46, no. 7 (1998): 922–926; and A Sehgal, "How Strictly do Dialysis Patients Want Their Advance Directives Followed?" *Journal of the American Medical Association* 267, no. 1 (1992): 59–63.

[38] Berger, DeRenzo, and Schwartz, 48.

[39] D Sulmasy, M Hughes, R Thompson, A Astrow, P Terry, and M Nolan, "How Would Terminally Ill Patients Have Others Make Decisions for Them in the Event of Decisional Incapacity?" *Journal of The American Geriatrics Society* 55, (2007): 1981–88.

apply. For example, she may have also stipulated that in the event she could no longer read, due to cognitive impairment, she does not wish to receive any more vision tests. Mrs. Black always hated having the drops put into her eyes. Probably this is a wish that could be seen to be applicable to her current situation. Another option (not mutually exclusive with the first) would be to reconsider the treatment refusal wish in the context of a best interest standard. It is reasonable, I think, to override her wish on the basis of it contravening her current interests; at least in Ontario, however, departing from wishes requires an application to the Consent and Capacity Board.

I think the second option, applying a best interest standard, is what makes more sense. In fact, the research supports this view. SDMs *often* do not follow advance directive wishes made by patients.[40] Additionally, many SDMs feel uncomfortable in their roles because they worry they do not know enough of what the patients meant to convey when the wishes were documented. It is actually astonishing to learn how few individuals have actually discussed their wishes at all with their SDMs.[41] Understandably, this often leaves the SDMs feeling inept about what to do. Rather than make a mistake, often their anxiety drives them to err on the side of caution, which, paradoxically, often results in patients having more treatments consented to, not less.[42]

(e) There are additional problems that arise within the context of SDM decision-making. Earlier I mentioned that SDMs tend to be family members or close friends of the patients. This piece of information is not surprising because they are the ones who tend to know the patients the best. They are also the ones whose own interests are likely to become the most entangled with those of the patients because of their close relationships. It can be difficult for them to separate out their own interests from those of the patients, with the result that it is more challenging to identify, let alone resolve, any conflicts of interests that arise. This particular dynamic is widespread. We have already discussed the myriad of interests that were operating among the patient, their family, and the team. It was possible that Brie's interests to keep her father alive were in conflict with those of her father and also in conflict with those of her brother. The

---

[40] Jox, 81–82. One of his empirical studies demonstrates that current nonverbal behavior has a higher impact on SDMs' treatment decisions than the patient's previously stated preferences.

[41] Carole Cohen, "Surrogate Decision Making: Special Issues in Geriatric Psychiatry," *Canadian Journal of Psychiatry* 49, no. 7 (July 2004): 454.

[42] This is also because we are mainly addressing advance directives with treatment refusal wishes (with the exception of receiving pain medication). If SDMs are not confident about how to interpret wishes of treatment refusal, there is a good likelihood that treatments that pertain to the respective wishes will not be refused. Hence, the patients end up getting what, at the time of writing the directive, was refused. For more information about SDMs defaulting to a position of requesting more treatment, not less, as a means to assuage their own moral distress in the face of uncertainty, see Ursula Brown, Aanand Naik, Laurence McCullough, "Reconceptualizing the Experience of Surrogate Decision Making: Reports vs Genuine Decisions, *Annals of Family Medicine* 7, no. 3 (May/June 2009): 249–253.

complexity of this case was further heightened by the fact that there were two SDMs.

The fact that conflicts of interests are likely to emerge should not be miscon-strued as necessarily a bad thing. They are borne out of caring, close ties that also render these SDMs to be in a privileged position in terms of access to intimate beliefs, wishes, and values of the patients. Nonetheless, these sorts of conflicts have the effect of creating tremendous moral distress among all involved. I have experienced many consultations where I have witnessed SDMs to be riddled with angst about how to manage the conflicting interests in tandem with intense emotionality. On more than one occasion, I have questioned the morality of subjecting patients' loved ones to this almost impossible task.

(f) Healthcare professionals play an important role in relation to the SDMs who are making decisions. We saw in the case of Mr. White that the practitioners natu-rally incline to a best interest approach, at least in part. I have also witnessed SDMs seemingly making choices contrary to the treatment wishes in directives and practitioners who require support to challenge them. Sometimes a SDM will want to make a decision that mainly favors another family member's inter-ests. I recall a son struggling to make a decision about whether or not to consent to life-saving treatment for his father who was very ill, and the effect of the treatment would be to possibly extend his life for a few months. The son was very concerned about the welfare of his mother, who had been stellar in support of her husband during his past 5 years of ill health. She was exhausted, stressed, and frail looking. The son wanted to go against the treatment (and not honor his father's advance directive) so that his mother could be relieved of her exhaust-ing caregiver role.

To summarize, in general, some SDMs and healthcare professionals do not always adhere to the legal hierarchy of decision-making standards[43]. They require support to do so. With regard to SDMs specifically, often the wishes are not understood with enough clarity for the SDMs to feel comfortable about providing consent to their application, in which case, thy are left to rely on their own interpretation of values and beliefs. Even when believed to be understood, SDMs, own interests sometimes become entangled with those of the patients', and one of the most dominating interests might be to keep the patients alive, so that the SDMs can forestall their own emotional loss. In addition, it is counter-intuitive not to consider patients' best interests, and this is one of the main reasons that the wishes contained in advance directives are not always complied with. The obligation of the SDMs to consider the applicability of the advance directive wishes to the current situation is a challenging one. SDMs are often unclear about what this clause actually means, and therefore there is lack of consistency with its interpretation. SDMs, with best intentions, may apply a best interest standard when attempting to fulfill this obligation.

In regard to the case of Mr. White, given that there was so much ambiguity about whether or not he met the criteria for informed consent for medical decision-

---

[43] Berger, DeRenzo and Schwartz, 48.

making, the role of his children became unclear as well, at least in terms of legal authority. There was much confusion about if and when they ought to have been assuming the substitute decision-making role, as well as there being divergent ideas about the veracity of their father's advance directive and even the interpretations and application of his wishes.

This case poignantly illustrates how challenging it is when there is more than one SDM involved. It also highlights the disposition, discussed earlier, either to intuitively favor the exclusive use of a best interest standard or, at a minimum, to integrate it with the values that are known.

Concluding Remarks

The case of Mr. White was the most complex one for me from an ethics point of view, among the three I have presented in this book.

One reason for this was that, from a legal point of view, many of the relevant issues were sitting in the borderline, the gray zone, so to speak. His competence was considered to be teetering at the legal margin for most of the time. It was debatable if his substitute decision-makers were entitled to partake in that role (contingent upon their father's capacity levels) or were overstepping their legal boundaries of voicing their directions as family members. We faced the issue about whether or not we should have been referring to his advance directive or, instead, his current wishes. Given how recently Mr. White had written his advance directive and that he was already experiencing mild dementia and the early effects of a brain tumor, on balance his advance directive probably was better informed than had that not been the case. It also seemed to make sense to consider it as a very recent capable wish, in tandem with his current wishes.

Since we could not easily situate ourselves within the context of the law, on one side or another, at least with the issues above, we straddled both sides. While my initial sense was that we were "all over the legal and moral map" with this case, I came to feel that our process was more rigorous, more integrating of a fuller person view. We employed as many approaches as we could. We used all the information we could. We referred to Mr. White's advance directive. We respected his current wishes too, though it is questionable if we should have done that to a greater degree. We looked to his best interests as well as to the values he seemed to hold dear. We considered the information imparted to us by the children. Much of this seemed to make intuitive sense. And I think this case demonstrated that the nuances and complexities of real-life clinical situations demand something "bigger" than the over-simplified approach of applying a lone legal standard.

According to the law, an advance directive is *not* the same as consent to a treatment; it is merely the expression of a wish. Therefore it does not need to meet medical standards of informed consent. The capacity to *express a wish* is distinguished from the capacity to make a *specific treatment decision* under the controlling case law. Informed consent in the context of signing a legal document is different than in the context of consenting to treatment, because it does not have to address risks and benefits particular to the treatment—not even if treatments or lack of treatments are listed or implied in the document itself. This level of consent is merely supposed to address questions of capacity, voluntariness, fraud, and undue influence. If the directive expresses treatment instructions, those instructions are the basis upon which the SDMs are obliged to give or refuse consent. There is, however, an obligation to examine the "quality" of the directive itself when there is information challenging whether the person understood what it meant or whether or not the person was (legally) capable at the time.[44]

Naturally, this contributes to the reasonable concerns about the legal standard that is applied to advance directives. First, while the capacity required to complete a directive is lower than that which is legally required to consent to treatment, there are no precise legal criteria in place, to my knowledge, that provide a definition by which we may judge how much lower it should be. Second, if the author of a directive specifies treatment instructions, it is incumbent upon the SDMs to ensure that they are acted upon, conditional upon their applicability to the current situation. If this condition is met, then the SDMs are obliged to consent.[45] On what basis ought the SDMs to decide if they should consent? It seems to me that consent is contingent only upon the directive being perceived by the SDMs to be applicable to the current situation. I take that to mean that the conditions stipulated in the directive match the current ones. When the author wrote the directive, there was no requirement to meet the treatment standards for informed consent, since the directive was merely the expression of a wish. If the SDMs are legally obliged to give informed consent on behalf of incapable patients, where in this process is the requirement of fulfillment of criteria for informed consent to occur? It was not a legal requirement of the author of the directive. Perhaps the requirement that the SDMs make a determination about whether the conditions stipulated in the directive match those occurring in the present entails that the SDMs be legally obliged to understand and appreciate the risks of the medical treatment now.

Suppose that it is within the SDMs' role to do so. Suppose further that the SDMs will be viewing this duty from the perspective of the patient having declined treatment. What information would be useful to them, other than applicability? Any weighing of consequences, risks, and benefits in relation to refusal of the treatment is first of all moot, because the patients already expressed their wishes to forego the treatment; the rationale for so doing is now practically irrelevant. If the SDMs are to give informed consent or refusal, then what is this based on? I think the answer is the applicability "standard." Clearly, it violates the spirit of the law for the SDMs to consider current risks and benefits in relation to the wishes expressed in the directives, because this approach would be a fresh exercise of autonomy, or best interests, or both. The point is that the SDMs are not giving informed consent, at least not in

---

[44] I am thankful to Mark Handelman, former vice chairperson of the Ontario Consent and Capacity Board, for apprising me of this legal distinction.

[45] We are assuming the patients were legally capable when they wrote the directive and that it was their most recent capable expressed wishes.

the way we are meant to apply it, from a legal perspective. The only other option is for an SDM to give informed consent to a plan of treatment, which is permitted in Ontario.

What is the applicability "test" supposed to do? Allow me to speculate.

The advance directive arose in large part as a backlash against medical paternalism or, in any case, the fear of medical paternalism. It was time to put medical treatment decision-making into the hands of the patients. As long as you could understand the relevant information and appreciate the benefits, risks, and consequences of a proposed treatment, you could make your own decision, *regardless of your reasons* (or lack thereof). The advance directive was a mechanism to do so now in contemplation of a future time of incapacity to do so.

When I say that if I can no longer recognize my family due to an irreversible condition or disease and I develop an illness, do not treat me; my reasons for stating these particular wishes are irrelevant. They are just as valid, legally, if they are based upon nonsense. I have no obligation to disclose them. There may not even be any relationship between the conditions or factors I state. They might just happen to be coexisting, independent of any meaning to one another. As soon as there is an attempt at speculation or inference-making, the whole point of autonomy, upon which the advent of the advance directive is based, is corrupted.

According to this "autonomy" account, I suggest it would make more sense for the document to stand alone, so to speak, without any SDM. The patient makes a decision (albeit uninformed, most likely), and if we believe in noninterference, we leave it be. The practitioner and/or other team members could render a confirmation if the conditions as stated in the directive are in existence today. If I cannot recognize my family members and if I have developed an illness that I earlier specified as calling for nontreatment, then, do not treat me, period. I would, however, rephrase the clause to read, "if the current situation is applicable to the wish" rather than the other way around. The task of determining applicability is not necessarily simple. There will be some uncomfortable squirming relative to the definition of recognition, duration of time expected, etc. But the wish should remain unexamined. As soon as the SDM tries to address the applicability question in the context of the wish, then reason, inference, and all kinds of other intrusions occur, borne out of concern or welfare for the patient.

The applicability step provides the wiggle room for a best interest standard to be smuggled in. But why arrange things so that this needs to be smuggled in under the cover of the applicability clause? We tend to naturally be interested in our own and other's welfare. Owing to poor preparation and a radically permissive legal constraint, at every possible opportunity, the advance directive is being sabotaged by its own authors, who expect their welfare to be considered by the SDMs, and by healthcare practitioners, who are by turns morally, legally, and professionally obliged to act benevolently.

It is hard to make sense out of the idea that an advance directive is a mere wish, of a sort not governed by constraints of informed consent, when the wishes it expresses are for treatments that would be governed by informed consent where they requested immediately and categorically. Arguably, the current capacity standard required to make treatment wishes is higher than that required to be legally capable to execute a directive. Nowhere, however, can I locate any legal information more specific than what I have just written.

Perhaps it could be argued, however, that the consent required of the SDM is *not* to be understood in the context of medical treatment decision-making but instead as that required to enforce the application of his advance directive as a legal document (not in reference specifically to its contents, which happen to speak to medical treatment directives). This argument is unconvincing to the extent that consent to apply the advance directive implies consent to the contents within it. And that, in turn, seems linked to the question of the state under which the author wrote the advance directive in the first place. Restricting the SDM's freedom to selectively apply or interpret the *contents* of the directive makes the most sense in the cases where it is clearest that such selectivity impinges on the author's autonomy, as expressed in his carefully considered written choices. The argument for restriction is weakest precisely when it seems least plausible that the author carefully considered the contents of the directive, his medical choices, in the first place. In my opinion, the only way to resolve this concern is to ensure that either the author of the advance directive had previously met the standards required to consent to treatment or to ensure that the SDM will meet them now. I would argue for the former resolution over the latter one, given that the whole idea of the advance directive was to ensure that autonomous wishes (as understood from within a legal framework) of the previously capable patient would be accorded to the future incapable patient. The autonomous prior capable wishes of the person who wrote the advance directive are, at a minimum, compromised if not nonexistent without informed medical treatment decision-making. Hence, it is significant that the prospects for an advance directive meeting the relevant standards are so poor, as I have already argued.

Sources

Benaroyo, Lazare and Guy Widdershoven. "Competence in Mental Health Care: a Hermeneutic Perspective." *Health Care Analysis* 12, no. 4 (December 2004): 297.

Berger, T., Evan G. DeRenzo, and Jack Schwartz. "Surrogate Decision Making: Reconciling Ethical Theory and Clinical Practice." *Annals of Internal Medicine*, no. 149 (2008): 48–53.

Brown, Ursula, Aanand Naik, and Lurence McCullough. "Reconceptualizing the Experience of Surrogate Decision Making: Reports vs. Genuine Decisions" *Annals of Family Medicine* 7, no. 3 (May/June 2009): 249–253.

Cohen, Carole A. "Surrogate Decision Making: Special Issues in Geriatric Psychiatry." *Canadian Journal of Psychiatry* 49, no. 7 (July 2004): 454–457.

Fellows, L.K. "Competency and Consent in Dementia." *Journal of the American Geriatrics Society* 46, no. 7 (1998): 922–926.

Health Care (Consent) and Care Facility (Admission) Act, R.S.B.C. Health Care (Consent) and Care Facility (Admission) Act, R.S.B.C. 1996, c.

Jox, Ralf. "Revocation of Advance Directives." In *Advance Directives*, edited by P. Lack, N. Biller-Andorno and S. Brauer. New York: Springer Press, 2014.

Olick, Robert S. "On the Scope and Limits of Advance Directives and Prospective Autonomy." In *Advance Directives*, edited by P. Lack, N. Biller-Andorno and S. Brauer. New York: Springer Press, 2014.

Sehgal A. "How Strictly do Dialysis Patients Want Their Advance Directives Followed?" *Journal of the American Medical Association* 267, no. 1 (1992): 59–63.

Sulmasy, D., Hughes, M., Thompson, T., Astrow, A., Terry, P. and Nolan, M. "How Would Terminally Ill Patients Have Others Make Decisions for Them in the Event of Decisional Incapacity?" *Journal of The American Geriatrics Society* 55, (2007): 1981–88.

Chapter 5
Conclusions

Advance directives came into existence based upon good intentions. Generally, the idea is to project medical treatment wishes into a future time of potential incapacity when treatment decisions might need to be made.

My experience as an ethicist, working in a number of healthcare facilities in Ontario, Canada, that provide medical treatment to patients with Alzheimer's dementia, portrays a range of significant concerns that arise out of the use of advance directives, at least in terms of how they are currently being used. What I have aimed to do in this book is identify and analyze some of the more prominent clinical ethics concerns that arise in the context of case studies. I then turned to the literature to seek ways of clearly understanding the problems that arose and potential practical assistance in mitigating the problems. The literature on this topic is quite robust, and all kinds of theoretical issues are identified, particularly in the epistemological and ontological realms; I have tried to distil some of the more useful elements of the literature to apply to these cases and these concerns. What I have concluded is that the use of advance directives with the Alzheimer's dementia population, *as it is currently used*, is fraught with problems that are mainly irresolvable. They are identified below. Some arise out of faulty premises upon which the notion of the advance directive was initially built.

1. The dominant conception about Alzheimer's dementia is that it is a disease of horrific tragedy and necessarily leads to "loss of personhood." You become less and less of who you were, apparently in ways that matter a great deal. The continuous belief in this portrayal of Alzheimer's plays a very significant role in the devaluing of persons with dementia and has all kinds of negative consequences, both obvious and subtle, when it comes to how we care for and respect persons with dementia. The negative stereotype of Alzheimer's is often at the root of why people write directives that state their desires to forego treatment if and when dementia strikes. It can be especially problematic to have such a directive if the person with dementia is generally happy as we witnessed in the case of Mrs. Black.

M. Sokolowski, *Dementia and the Advance Directive*,
https://doi.org/10.1007/978-3-319-72083-8_5

2. I think it is problematic that the legal concept of autonomy employs a very narrow definition and explicit criteria that have to do with autonomous decision-making and specifically with informed consent (itself a specialized legal notion in this context). Rather than considering directly what is important to being an autonomous person, this standard concerns itself with legal criteria for making an autonomous decision. For an independent, person without dementia, this approach may have made sense. For persons with dementia who cannot necessarily meet the legal standard, it fails to accord with their preferences or states of mind and undermines their participation in processes where medical treatment decision-making may have very significant results for them. What this did for the patients who I profiled in this book was to continuously subject them to the process of determining whether or not they could meet the standard of informed consent, one treatment decision episode at a time. The chances of them being able to meet the threshold, raised in proportion to perceived risks, were predictably very slim and even potentially slimmer as the kinds of decisions that matter the most were presented. When deemed incapable of making a current autonomous decision, the default standard became the advance directive (if considered to be the most recent capable wish). This problem arises in part because of the mistaken assumption that *a* legal standard appropriate at most to a particular range of circumstances can successfully be applied to complex and nuanced clinical situations that persons are embedded within. It fails to take into consideration the context from within which these standards are to be applied. It privileges a very narrow account of autonomy, one I have described as "hyper-cognitivist," which does not cohere with what it means to be an autonomous person in a fuller sense and what it means to respectfully care for human beings who have dementia. The relational aspect of autonomy is not reflected in the principle of autonomy as it is represented in medical contexts.

3. An additional and related problem is to assume that most people with dementia (beyond the very early stage) could not be autonomous. This had to do with the conflation already mentioned between an important but limited notion of autonomous decision-making (being able to make an informed decision) and being autonomous, as well as the conflation between autonomy and capable. If a person with dementia could be autonomous in some degree, then an advance directive would play a much more circumscribed role than the one it is typically taken to play. This issue that the person with dementia is assumed to be nonautonomous does not fit with what I experience in clinical situations. Persons are larger than their abilities to make informed decisions. Nor is there consistency among practitioners in terms of how their determinations are arrived at.

4. One faulty premise underlying the conception of an advance directive is that one can actually project his or her own treatment wishes into the future; another is that doing so would remedy the initial problem of the patient with dementia not being able to express autonomous treatment wishes. This concept of applying previous wishes to circumstances in the future of a person with dementia is known as "precedent autonomy." The idea of the directive was founded on the assumption of legal and moral equivalence between everyday (contemporaneous)

autonomy and precedent autonomy. Largely due to unknown future circumstances and associated lack of information, coupled with predictive moral imagination fallibility, in the vast majority of cases, the authors of directives are neither able nor *could* be able (largely due to reasons extrinsic to themselves) to understand the pertinent information they would need nor to appreciate the consequences of their refusal or acceptance of treatment. Due to these epistemic problems, as well as to the problem of irreversibility of decisions, I suggest that precedent autonomy is not morally (nor should legally be considered) equivalent to contemporaneous autonomy. In fact, the notion of precedent autonomy being foundational to the concept of the advance directive is at best, quite weak, and only in very selected cases could it deserve much moral weight.

Even without these very fundamental problems involving autonomy, there are always practical implementation problems related to trying to apply subjective interpretations to the instructions in an advance directive. There are very few situations where an advance directive could be said to have met the requirements of informed consent. In the case of Mr. White, I argued that his directive was less problematic than were the others in terms of predictability, but nonetheless problems did occur, and this type of situation was quite exceptional anyway.

Unless a different standard was to be established and/or a reconceptualization of the notion of autonomy was adopted, I see no solution being possible within the current paradigm.

5. My analysis of each case included the question of whether the directive met the standard of informed consent, given the alleged equivalence between precedent autonomy and contemporaneous autonomy (proven in reality to be mythical). I believed this question to be necessarily relevant.

However, the Canadian province of Ontario does *not* require that an advance directive meet the legal standard of informed consent. While initially this information may seem to be solving one problem—we no longer have to worry about the directive meeting the informed consent standard because it is not legally expected to—a more dire concern is raised. In addition to the confusion that arises in terms of the conceptualization of the directive and its intended use, we learn that *something less* than the standard of informed consent is considered acceptable to use because *wishes* are being advanced, *not treatment decisions*. It is *not just* that the bar has been lowered (apparently the test for capacity to execute an advance directive is much lower than the test for capacity to make a specific treatment decision); there is a lack of robust objective standards in place. I do not know what the criteria would amount to in terms of reaching a conclusion that the author of the directive is incapable to formulate a directive, let alone know how we could know that such a situation even existed. A very significant problem arises in the context of the legal requirement to act upon the wishes in the directive (outside of certain exclusionary factors such as proof of incapacity at the time the directive was written or the SDM refusing to give consent because the wishes are not applicable to the current situation) under less-than-ideal circumstances. After all, just about anything could qualify as a wish. What we do know with more certainty is what standard is not being met and that a standard lower than that of informed consent is considered acceptable. I venture that we are likely no better off than we are when we believe that we ought to be meeting the standard of informed consent (when in fact rarely could we be).

6. It is problematic to assume that having an SDM to interpret the directive and provide the requisite informed consent generally adds merit. Also, we have discussed research findings that conclude that it is not unusual for an SDM to apply the best interest standard when contemplating whether or not to give consent to directives, either as the sole standard or in conjunction with an autonomy standard. When SDMs apply the best interest standard, he or she might be privileging particular kinds of interests over others and not necessarily the patient's interests over others. SDMs do not always follow even relatively clearly expressed treatment wishes, for a variety of reasons. We also know from research that physicians and/or other team members do not necessarily intend to follow what the patient or the SDM expects. There is potentially tremendous subjectivity, variation, and inconsistency occurring with regard to the conceptualization of the advance directive, how its contents gets interpreted, its intended and actual use, and how and if it gets applied.

   We also learned that this would be a mistake to assume that the author of the directive behaves in a more predictable fashion. It would not be exceptional for him or her to neither expect nor even want the directive to be perceived as definitive. Some do wish for it to be literally complied with. Others want their interests at the time of incapacity to prevail, some interests taking precedence over others, while others expect a combination of directive wishes and current best interests to be determining. Rarely, however, are these expectations or wishes known to the SDM. Even if they were, they would not necessarily prove to be the current expectations or wishes of the patient with dementia. By chance, however, a previous wish (of a formerly capable person) that the same person with dementia currently continues to hold might be consented to by the respective SDM. After all, there are only two possible outcomes, consent and refusal.

7. As it is currently legally defined by Ontario's *Health Care Consent Act*, the best interests principle seems to be more defensible as a standard of decision-making for persons with dementia than is the legal default principle (see Appendix), which requires that the SDM give or refuse consent in harmony with an applicable previously expressed *capable wish*. The best interests principle seems to make intuitive sense (either on its own or in conjunction with the default principle) to many SDMs, team members, and patients alike, as it incorporates current wishes of the dementia patient as well as their best interests as determined objectively (or intersubjectively) by SDMs and the medical team. So at least there is some reference to the person with dementia having potential merit ascribed to present interests, wishes, and/or values. This is a far cry from, and a great improvement upon, what the default principle requires, with its overarching stipulation that "if the SDM knows of a wish applicable to the circumstances that the incapable person expressed while capable and after attaining 16 years of age, the person shall give or refuse consent in accordance with the wish." As defined in Ontario, the best interests principle seems to be founded upon a much more realistic, nuanced, and complex picture of what it means to be a person, above

and beyond the rational attributes legally associated with capacity or "capability," and allows for the consideration that a person with dementia is a person who currently has values, interests, and wishes. The potential implications for moral actions in terms of how we care for persons with dementia are worthy of further exploration.

8. While advance directives often create more problems than they are worth, a directive completed by someone in close temporal proximity to an event or illness (that will render their immediate interests, values, and wishes unknowable) is likely to have some merit, provided the state was explicitly described and the wishes were well articulated. In such a situation, an advance directive would likely be a better option than not having any idea about what to do. A person in a comatose state would be in such a situation, and the relevance of the advance directive increases to the extent that the person in question is not known by anyone in the position of needing to make a medical decision. Interestingly enough, I imagine an advance directive might prove to be its most useful when someone is a complete stranger to us, one who cannot communicate through any means, wishes, interests, or values. A stranger in a coma is the most likely type of person to potentially accrue some benefit from a directive. If this same stranger does not happen to have a directive, then from a legal point of view, he or she will have decisions made according to the principle of best interests.

   But persons with dementia are not moral strangers to us, unless we choose to treat them as such.

9. Finally, I wish to return to my initial statement that the intentions behind the creation of the advance directive were honorable. There is something rightly important about giving voice to wishes of a person with dementia with regard to consent or refusal of medical treatments being currently offered. Aside from chance, I estimate that rarely would end up happening through the usual way we have been utilizing advance directives with the dementia population. Nonetheless perhaps the advance directive's greatest virtue of all is the role it is playing in motivating healthcare professionals to embrace the intention of honoring the wishes, interests, and values of persons with dementia but to do so through engagement in *advance care planning*[1] with their patients as an *ongoing process* and in a *proactive* way.

Source

Seymour, Jane and Home, Gillian. "Advance Care Planning for the end of life: an overview." In *Advance Care Planning in End of Life Care*, edited by K. Thomas and B. Lobo. Oxford: Oxford University Press, 2011, 16–27.

---

[1] For a comprehensive overview of advance care planning see Jane Seymour and Gillian Horne, "Advance Care Planning for the end of life: an overview" in Advance Care Planning in End of Life Care, ed. Keri Thomas and Ben Lobo (Oxford: Oxford University Press, 2011), 16–27.

Chapter 6
Recommendations

Clinical Recommendations

1. An advance directive ought to be explicitly considered as one piece of information among many about a person's intentions and/or preferences. It is not the sole determinant of settling any medical treatment decisions.
2. Because an advance directive document is at best a weak example of the principle of autonomy, treatment wishes in an advance directive should not be construed as equivalent to, or having the same self-determination status as, treatment wishes made "in real time" by the patient.
3. Many people with dementia will be capable of holding values, wishes, and interests that matter to them. On this view, they ought to be considered to be at least borderline or partially autonomous, and medical treatment decisions should be made that cohere with them, whenever possible.
4. A relational view of autonomy ought to be preferred to the traditional (independent) view of autonomy in healthcare facilities. In particular a relational view of autonomy holds that one's choices inherently reflect or depend on others' values, interests, abilities, and wishes. Hence patients with dementia should receive the support required from others in the expression of their values, wishes, and interests when needed.
5. Currently held and known values, interests and wishes of the dementia patient should override an advance directive. When current-but-unclear expressions (or indirect indications) of wishes from an inconsistent, confused, and inarticulate patient are weighed against past-but-seemingly-clear expressions of wishes in the advance directive (the clarity of which can be illusory, once one takes seriously how ill-informed the writing process is), the principle of autonomy should lead us to err on the side of seeking to honor people's tendency and right to *change* with respect to what they feel, what they prefer, what they value.
6. A directive that is very recent and does not seem to have been made obsolete by changes in the patient's statements or attitudes/responses to treatment can be

© Springer International Publishing AG 2018
M. Sokolowski, *Dementia and the Advance Directive*,
https://doi.org/10.1007/978-3-319-72083-8_6

treated simply as a current expression of the patient's wishes. Then, in some imprecise but significant way, its status as a current expression (hence to be taken as an exercise of autonomy) degrades quickly with the passage of time or the onset of attitudes/behavior (e.g., general happiness) in tension with the content or presuppositions of the advance directive.

7. Autonomy of persons with dementia should be safeguarded independently of legal frameworks for establishing capacity. If this recommendation proves impractical or futile, then I recommend that we lower, not raise, the capacity threshold when the decisions in question matter most to the persons with dementia.

8. Healthcare organizations ought to develop guidelines and frameworks treating advance care planning as an ongoing process, as opposed to relying on a specific document such as an advance directive.

9. All stakeholders, including patients, substitute decision-makers, staff members, and significant others, should receive ongoing education about the challenges and strengths of advance directives. In addition, empirical research indicating that SDMs do not necessarily follow the wishes of advance directives ought to be shared as well.

10. Laying out a support structure and decision framework is a far more legitimate undertaking for a pre-dementia advance directive than attempting to specify precise treatment preferences and anti-preferences. Decision-making frameworks ought to support transparency of all stakeholders' values, conflicts, and interests and address how conflicts should attempt to be resolved. Advance directives ought to focus more on how the SDM should make decisions.

11. Making choices on behalf of a person with diminished independence is *very difficult*. I recommend that we adopt a working-group approach which capitalizes on a variety of perspectives. The SDM hopefully can contribute valuable knowledge about the patient's longer-term interests and dispositions; staff members bring medical expertise, as well as knowledge related to current states of the patient's mind and seeming preferences; and the ethicist can facilitate a moral deliberation process.

12. Ongoing plan of care reviews ought to include the identification of current (and/or potential future) conflicts of interests between all stakeholders (both within and external to the teams) and provide guidelines and structures for how conflicts of interest can be dealt with. It is important that the existence of conflicts of interest be normalized and a proactive approach be undertaken in terms of identification and potential resolution whenever possible.

13. The prevalent conception of Alzheimer's as a disease that destroys personhood ought to be actively challenged.

Policy Recommendations

1. From a legal point of view, a best interest standard ought to be applied to an advance directive. A "best interest" standard is more robust as it captures the range of current and past values, interests, and wishes. Generally, those more currently held and/or expressed by the patient usurp those of the past.
2. The default position is that the patient with dementia is autonomous and holds values, interests, and wishes that are meaningful to him or her.
3. Develop guidelines for ongoing advance care planning processes that require open, reflective, and transparent frameworks of decision-making that best reflect (to the extent possible) the current (and future as appropriate) values, needs, and wishes of the patient with dementia.
4. Consent to treatment acts, such as Ontario's *Health Care Consent Act, 1996* ought to be redrafted in such a way as to ensure that people with dementia can participate directly or indirectly in decision-making, to the extent possible. Every attempt should be made to elicit patients' understanding and appreciation in ways that are enabling to the patients and may include engaging other persons to assist the patients to do so, as appropriate.
5. Substitute decision-makers ought to be educated about their role and responsibilities and must express their willingness to undertake their role. In particular, they should be included in ongoing advance care planning (with patient permission), whenever possible.
6. Healthcare organizations should assume responsibility to ensure that all stakeholders are briefed on the legal and clinical guidelines related to advance care planning.

Appendix

Ontario's *Health Care Consent Act, 1996*[1]

Purposes

1. The purposes of this Act are:

   (a) To provide rules with respect to consent to treatment that applies consistently in all settings

   (b) To facilitate treatment, admission to care facilities, and personal assistance services for persons lacking the capacity to make decisions about such matters

   (c) To enhance the autonomy of persons for whom treatment is proposed, persons for whom admission to a care facility is proposed, and persons who are to receive personal assistance services by:

      (i) Allowing those who have been found to be incapable to apply to a tribunal for a review of the finding

      (ii) Allowing incapable persons to request that a representative of their choice be appointed by the tribunal for the purpose of making decisions on their behalf concerning treatment, admission to a care facility, or personal assistance services

      (iii) Requiring that wishes with respect to treatment, admission to a care facility, or personal assistance services, expressed by persons while capable and after attaining 16 years of age, be adhered to

   (d) Promote communication and understanding between health practitioners and their patients or clients.

---

[1] www.e-laws.gov.on.ca/html/statutes/english/elaws_statutes_96h02_e.htm

© Springer International Publishing AG 2018
M. Sokolowski, *Dementia and the Advance Directive*,
https://doi.org/10.1007/978-3-319-72083-8

(e) Ensure a significant role for supportive family members when a person lacks the capacity to make a decision about a treatment, admission to a care facility, or a personal assistance service.

(f) Permit intervention by the Public Guardian and Trustee only as a last resort in decisions on behalf of incapable persons concerning treatment, admission to a care facility, or personal assistance services (1996, c. 2, Sched. A, s. 1)

Consent to Treatment

No Treatment Without Consent

10. (1) A health practitioner who proposes a treatment for a person shall not administer the treatment and shall take reasonable steps to ensure that it is not administered, unless:

    (a) He ort she is of the opinion that the person is capable with respect to the treatment, and the person has given consent.

    (b) He or she is of the opinion that the person is incapable with respect to the treatment, and the person's substitute decision-maker has given consent on the person's behalf in accordance with this Act (1996, c. 2, Sched. A, s. 10 (1)).

Elements of Consent

11. (1) The following are the elements required for consent to treatment:

    1. The consent must relate to the treatment.
    2. The consent must be informed.
    3. The consent must be given voluntarily.
    4. The consent must not be obtained through misrepresentation or fraud (1996, c. 2, Sched. A, s. 11 (1)).

Informed Consent

(2) A consent to treatment is informed if, before giving it,

    (a) The person received the information about the matters set out in subsection (3) that a reasonable person in the same circumstances would require in order to make a decision about the treatment.

    (b) The person received responses to his or her requests for additional information about those matters (1996, c. 2, Sched. A, s. 11 (2)).

Same

(3) The matters referred to in subsection (2) are:

1. The nature of the treatment
2. The expected benefits of the treatment
3. The material risks of the treatment
4. The material side effects of the treatment
5. Alternative courses of action
6. The likely consequences of not having the treatment (1996, c. 2, Sched. A, s. 11 (3))

Capacity

Capacity Depends on Treatment

15. (1) A person may be incapable with respect to some treatments and capable with respect to others (1996, c. 2, Sched. A, s. 15 (1)).

Capacity Depends on Time

(2) A person may be incapable with respect to a treatment at one time and capable at another (1996, c. 2).

Principles for Giving or Refusing Consent

21. (1) A person who gives or refuses consent to a treatment on an incapable person's behalf shall do so in accordance with the following principles:

1. If the person knows of a wish applicable to the circumstances that the incapable person expressed while capable and after attaining 16 years of age, the person shall give or refuse consent in accordance with the wish.
2. If the person does not know of a wish applicable to the circumstances that the incapable person expressed while capable and after attaining 16 years of age, or if it is impossible to comply with the wish, the person shall act in the incapable person's best interests (1996, c. 2, Sched. A, s. 21 (1)).

Best Interests

(2) In deciding what the incapable person's best interests are, the person who gives or refuses consent on his or her behalf shall take into consideration:

(a) The values and beliefs that the person knows the incapable person held when capable and believes he or she would still act on if capable

(b) Any wishes expressed by the incapable person with respect to the treatment that are not required to be followed under paragraph 1 of subsection (1)

(c) The following factors:

1. Whether the treatment is likely to:

   i. Improve the incapable person's condition or well-being
   ii. Prevent the incapable person's condition or well-being from deteriorating
   iii. Reduce the extent to which, or the rate at which, the incapable person's condition or well-being is likely to deteriorate

2. Whether the incapable person's condition or well-being is likely to improve, remain the same, or deteriorate without the treatment

3. Whether the benefit the incapable person is expected to obtain from the treatment outweighs the risk of harm to him or her

4. Whether a less restrictive or less intrusive treatment would be as beneficial as the treatment that is proposed (1996, c. 2, Sched. A, s. 21 (2))

Index

The manufacturer's authorised representative in the EU is Springer
Nature Customer Service Centre GmbH, Europaplatz 3, 69115 Heidelberg,
Germany. If you have any concerns regarding our products, please
contact ProductSafety@springernature.com

Printed and bound by CPI Group (UK) Ltd, Croydon, CR0 4YY

29/04/2026

02099619-0002